# TRADITIONAL CHINESE INTERNAL MEDICINE

*Xie Zhufan    Liao Jiazhen*

FOREIGN LANGUAGES PRESS    BEIJING

First Edition     1993

ISBN 7-119-01600-8

© Foreign Languages Press, Beijing, 1993
Published by Foreign Languages Press
24 Baiwanzhuang Road, Beijing 100037, China

Printed by Beijing Foreign Languages Printing House
19 Chegongzhuang Xilu, Beijing 100044, China

Distributed by China International Book Trading Corporation
35 Chegongzhuang Xilu, Beijing 100044, China
P.O. Box 399, Beijing, China

*Printed in the People's Republic of China*

# CONTENTS

# PART ONE

# CHAPTER I   THE THEORY OF *YIN-YANG*

*Yin* and *yang* were and still are two topographic terms used to designate the shady and the sunny sides of a hill, respectively. This can be illustrated by analysis of the Chinese characters 陰 (*yin*) and 陽 (*yang*) in modern script or 霒 (*yin*) and 昜 (*yang*) in ancient calligraphic style, which is still used on seals today. Either 阝 or 自 denotes a hill; 日 or ⊖ is a symbol of the sun, while 云 or 彡 a pictograph of a cloud. 昜 is composed of the horizon—and the sunshine 勿 . 仐 is a phonetic symbol indicating the sound of "yin." So it is not difficult to understand the original meaning of these two characters.

Since everything under the sun has two sides, the sunny and the shady, by extension of meaning *yin* and *yang* represent the two opposites of an object or a phenomenon. The theory of *yin-yang* as an ancient Chinese philosophy was used to explain changes in nature. According to this theory, all things and phenomena in the universe contain two opposite aspects, *yin* and *yang*, which are in conflict and at the same time interdependent. Thus, this theory represents the law of the unity of opposites. As relates to medicine, its main content can be summarized in the following points:

## I. The Opposition of *Yin* and *Yang*

First of all, *yin* and *yang* represent the basic properties of the two opposites. The most frequent uses of *yin* and *yang* in this sense in traditional medicine are listed in Table I-I.

**Table I-I. Classification of Properties of Objects or Phenomena According to *Yin-Yang***

|      | Space            | Mass—Energy  | Weight | Temperature  |
| ---- | ---------------- | ------------ | ------ | ------------ |
| Yin  | Interior—Lower   | Substantial  | Heavy  | Cold or Cool |
| Yang | Exterior—Upper   | Functional   | Light  | Hot or Warm  |

|      | Brightness | State                            | Time  |
| ---- | ---------- | -------------------------------- | ----- |
| Yin  | Dim        | Quiescent—Descending—Inhibited   | Slow  |
| Yang | Bright     | Moving—Ascending—Excited         | Rapid |

For example, the meridians running through the medial aspect of the limbs are called *yin* meridians, while those running through the lateral aspect of the limbs *yang* meridians. Among pathogenic factors, cold and damp are *yin* factors, while dryness and heat are *yang* factors. Dim yellow coloration of the skin and eyes, chronic in progress and accompanied by "cold" symptoms, is called *yin* jaundice, while bright yellow coloration of the skin and eyes, acute in onset and accompanied by fever or "heat" symptoms, is *yang* jaundice.

Although *yin* and *yang* give some information about the things they qualify, the

· 3

attribution is very general. Classification of the pathogenic factors into more details, such as wind, cold, damp, dryness, heat and fire, is more appropriate for clinical use than the gross groupings of *yin* factors and *yang* factors. Therefore, use of terms with *yin* and *yang* as attributives is avoided as much as possible in this book. However, among various pairs of opposites, the structural or material aspect of the human body which pertains to *yin* and the functional aspect which pertains to *yang* are a pair of opposites which are of utmost importance in physiology and pathology.

Just as some adjectives can function as nouns in English, *yin* and *yang* can also be used in a similar way. Thus, when we say kidney-*yin*, we actually refer to the structural materials of the kidneys, especially the essence stored in them; and when we say kidney-*yang*, we refer to its functions. In this sense *yin* and *yang* can hardly be totally replaced by other terms and are therefore widely used in the present writings of traditional Chinese medicine, including this book.

This discussion is limited only to terminology. As a philosophical theory of opposition, the concept of *yin-yang* pervades traditional Chinese medicine.

## II. Interdependence of *Yin* and *Yang*

Although *yin* and *yang* are in opposition to each other, they are mutually dependent. Neither *yin* nor *yang* can exist in isolation; without its opposite aspect, each loses the condition for its existence. For example, without "above," there would be no "below"; without "brightness," there would be no "darkness"; without "movement," there would be no "quiescence"; without "excitation," there would be no "inhibition." All the opposites exist together, just as the head and tail of a coin.

The application of the interdependence of *yin* and *yang* to medicine can be demonstrated by the interrelationship between essential substances (*yin*) and functional activities (*yang*). Substance is the basis of function, while function is the reflection of the existence of the substance and the motive force for the production of substance. Only when there are ample substances can the functional activities of the human body and its various systems be healthy. Only when the functional activities of various systems are sound, are they able to constantly produce substances. The coordination and harmonious equilibrium between substance and function, i.e., between *yin* and *yang*, is the vital guarantee for all physiological processes.

The interdependence of *yin* and *yang* is also used to represent pathological changes. Since *yin* and *yang* rely on each other for existence, impairment of *yin* impedes the generation of *yang*; impairment of *yang* impedes the generation of *yin*. For example, persistent impairment of the digestive function may lead to malnutrition and anemia — deficiency of *yin* caused by impairment of *yang*. Acute massive loss of blood may give rise to failure of peripheral circulation — impairment of *yang* due to deficiency of *yin*.

## III. The relative waxing and waning of *Yin* and *Yang*

The opposites in all objects and phenomena are in constant motion, one's growth resulting in the other's decline, one's advance marked by the other's retreat. The opposites maintain a normal process of development through this dynamic equilibrium. In the natural world the most obvious example is the change of seasons. From spring to summer the weather gets warmer and warmer — a waning of *yin* together with a waxing of *yang*. From autumn to winter the weather gets cool to cold — a waning of the *yang* together with a waxing of the *yin*.

This concept of the waxing and waning of *yin* and *yang* has also been applied to medicine in order to explain physiological activities and pathological changes. It is held that a person's life is a physiological process in constant motion and change which is reflected in the normal waxing and waning of *yin* and *yang*. For instance, functional activities (*yang*) consume nutrient substances (*yin*) — waning of *yin* with waxing of *yang*. Formation and storage of nutrient substances consume functional energy — waxing of *yin* with waning of *yang*.

Under normal conditions the waxing and waning of *yin* and *yang* remains within certain limits, reflecting the dynamic equilibrium of physiological processes.

When the relative balance of *yin* and *yang* is lost, disease occurs. Four common patterns of imbalance of *yin* and *yang* serve as the basic pathogenetic mechanisms of various diseases. They are 1) excess of *yin* with relative deficiency of *yang*; 2) excess of *yang* with relative deficiency of *yin*; 3) deficiency of *yin* with relative excess of *yang*; and 4) deficiency of *yang* with relative excess of *yin*. Of course, there may be other patterns, such as deficiency of both *yin* and *yang*, excess of both *yin* and *yang* and jumbled cases.

# CHAPTER II  THE STRUCTURE AND FUNCTIONS
## OF THE HUMAN BODY

Traditional Chinese medicine, shaped by philosophy and restricted by the historical conditions of the natural sciences, is quite different from modern Western medicine in its conception of the structure of the human body. One of the most outstanding features of this conception is that of the human body as an integral whole. All component parts, including organs and tissues, are considered with respect to the whole body and to their close interrelationships. However, individual parts are ill-defined, especially from the modern anatomical point of view. This makes traditional Chinese medicine a unique system, one that at times seems fantastic and always resists easy comprehension. It is noteworthy that during its long history of development, traditional Chinese medicine has undergone great improvements, yet little modification in the conception of the structure of the human body has occurred.

In fact, most of the traditional theories and principles are founded not upon anatomy but rather upon functional activities, either physiological or pathophysiological, and rely particularly heavily upon the notion of therapeutic effects. It should also be noted that all the traditional physiological and pathophysiological knowledge was not obtained by laboratory experimentation on isolated organs and systems but rather through the clinical observations of practitioners who viewed the human body as an organic whole.

In traditional Chinese medicine internal organs are the core structure of the functions of the human body. An internal organ in traditional Chinese medicine, also called *zang-fu* according to transliteration, refers to a comprehensive system of physiological functions rather than an anatomical entity. There are five *zang* organs: heart, liver, spleen, lungs and kidneys. There are six *fu* organs: small intestine, gall bladder, stomach, large intestine, urinary bladder and *sanjiao* (triple energizer)*. Generally speaking, *zang* organs are solid visceral organs, while *fu* organs are hollow, serving chiefly as passages for food, water and waste.

Physiologically, structural and functional connections exist among both the *zang* and *fu* organs. Each *zang* organ is particularly associated with a *fu* organ. They share functions and are connected by meridians, i.e., the heart and the small intestine, the liver and the gall bladder, the spleen and the stomach, the lungs and the large intestine and

---

*Sanjiao* (triple energizer) actually refers to the body cavities: the upper-*jiao* or upper energizer is the thoracic cavity in which the heart and lungs are situated; the middle-*jiao* or middle energizer is the upper abdominal cavity where the spleen and stomach lie; and the lower-*jiao* or lower energizer is the rest of the abdominal cavity containing the liver, kidneys, intestines and bladder. In some instances, each part of *sanjiao* can be used as a comprehensive name for the organs it contains, e.g., the middle-*jiao* can mean the spleen and stomach.

the kidneys and the urinary bladder.*

## I. The *Zang* organs

### 1. The heart

The heart, situated in the thoracic cavity (upper energizer) and covered by the pericardium for protection, controls the blood and houses the mind.

(1) Controlling blood and vessels. The beat of the heart sends blood circulating through the vessels to nourish the whole body. This concept is similar to that of Western medicine.

(2) Housing the mind. The heart governs mental activities, including spirit, consciousness, memory, thinking and sleep. This concept seems entirely different from the modern Western point of view, but semantic similarities can be easily found in the English language. For instance, to play something "by heart" means "from memory"; to "lose heart" means "to be discouraged"; "to take heart" means "to be confident." Thus, the word "heart" in daily English also connotes mental activities.

### 2. The liver

The liver is said to be a "viscus of temperament." Its main functions are storing blood, smoothing and regulating the flow of *qi* (vital energy) and blood, and controlling the tendons (muscular movements). They are also closely related to the eye, which is considered "the window of the liver."

(1) Being a "viscus of temperament." This metaphor indicates that, on the one hand, the liver is easily affected by temperamental or emotional factors, especially depression and anger, and on the other hand, irascibility or bad temper is one of the chief symptoms when the liver is diseased. This concept of the liver is apparently different from that of Western modern medicine. However, semantics may again give a clue as to the similarity between Chinese and Western culture. In English, the word "livery" or "liverish" has dual meaning, i.e., "suffering from liver trouble" and "irritable or of a hot temper."

(2) Storing blood. The liver stores blood and regulates the volume of circulating blood. This is roughly in accord with modern Western physiology. However, there exists a divergence of views. For instance, in traditional Chinese medicine infrequent, scanty or even suppressed menstruation is explained in most cases as a manifestation of insufficient blood storage of the liver; hematemesis precipitated by a fit of anger is usually taken as an example of the disordered blood-storage function of the liver.

(3) Smoothing and regulating the flow of *qi* and blood. *Qi* refers to the energy required for various functional activities, and the smooth flow of *qi* and blood is a prerequisite for maintaining normal functional activities. The liver smoothes and regulates the flow of *qi* and blood, promoting harmonious and unobstructed functional activities, including the following:

(a) Emotion. As mentioned above, the liver is closely related to emotional activities. Dysfunction of the liver with stagnant flow of *qi* may bring on depression. On the other hand, when the liver function is over-exercised, the patient becomes irritable and irascible.

(b) Digestion. The *qi* (energy) for digestive activities is particularly regulated by the

---

*Closely related to *sanjiao* is the pericardium, which is also considered a *zang* organ in another formulation of the *zang-fu* organs, but this is not emphasized in this book in order to avoid confusion.

liver. If the flow of *qi* is impeded in liver diseases, digestive disorders usually occur, such as belching, vomiting, abdominal distention and diarrhea.

(c) Bile secretion. Secretion of the bile, its storage in the gallbladder and discharge into the intestine are all related to the function of the liver in smoothing and regulating the flow of *qi*.

(d) Blood circulation. *Qi* is also the energy required for blood circulation. Depressed flow of *qi* may stagnate blood circulation. Obstruction of the flow of *qi* and blood is the most common cause of pain. Therefore, dysfunction of the liver is often accompanied by pain, particularly in the regions where the Liver Meridian passes, e.g., in the mammary, lateral pectoral, hypochondriac, lateral abdominal and inguinal regions.

(4) Controlling the "tendons" (muscular movements). In traditional Chinese medicine "tendon" refers to the mechanical elements of the locomotive system, the function of which is muscular movements and physical activities. When one is active, the musculature requires a supply of blood. Since the liver stores blood and sends it into circulation when it is required, thus nourishing the tendons. Therefore, it is said that the liver controls the function of the tendons, keeping them in a normal state of contraction or relaxation. In morbid conditions, impaired movements of the joints may be due to insufficient storage of blood in the liver. Abnormal muscular contractions, such as convulsions, opisthotonos, trismus and tremors, are usually attributed to dysfunction of the liver.

### 3. The spleen

The concept of the spleen in traditional Chinese medicine diverges even more from the modern concept. According to the classical description of the spleen in traditional anatomy, it includes the pancreas and is described as a "fatty appendage." Its main physiological functions are transporting and transforming water and food essence, reinforcing *qi*, keeping the blood flowing within the blood vessels and nourishing the muscles.

(1) Transporting and transforming water and food essence. This implies digestion of food and absorption and transmission of the nutrients to the heart and the lungs for nourishing the whole body. Since the spleen plays such a vital role, it is considered a source of essential substances for growth and development and forms the basis of a person's acquired constitution. If this function is impaired, anorexia, abdominal distension, diarrhea and malnutrition usually occur.

The spleen also monitors the absorption and transmission of fluids. That is why edema in some cases is attributed to dysfunction of the spleen.

(2) Reinforcing *qi*. *Qi*, especially acquired *qi*, derives from the nutrients absorbed as well as the oxygen inhaled. Therefore, the production of *qi* is closely related to the function of the spleen. When functioning soundly, the spleen provides sufficient nutrients for the production of *qi*, while an impaired spleen often leads to deficiency of *qi*.

(3) Keeping the blood flowing within the vessels. This prevents the circulating blood from extravasating. Impairment of this function usually gives rise to chronic hemorrhagic diseases.

(4) Nourishing the muscles. Here the word "muscle" implies the flesh of the muscles, the somatic element which gives the body its characteristic shape and physical strength. This is closely related to the function of the spleen in transforming and transmitting food

essence. If the spleen is impaired, especially over a long period of time, emaciation, lassitude and asthenia will result.

### 4. The lungs

The word "lungs" in traditional Chinese medicine has a broader connotation than that in Western medicine. The former includes the whole respiratory system, and even some functions other than respiration. The lungs dominate *qi*, control respiration, take charge of the skin and hair (resistance against disease of the body surface) and regulate water passages.

(1) Dominating *qi* (including respiration). The physiological *qi*, which serves as the dynamic force or energy for the functional activities of the human body, is formed by combining the clean air (oxygen) inhaled by the lungs and the food essence absorbed by the spleen. Thus, the lungs dominate *qi* in two ways: their respiratory function and their supply of oxygen for the formation of vital energy. Therefore, when the function of the lungs is insufficient, shortness of breath and general weakness result.

The function of the lungs includes dispersing and descending properties. "Dispersing" refers to the lungs' capacity to disseminate *qi* throughout the body, while "descending" refers to the sending down of fresh air (oxygen) through the air passage during inhalation. In lung diseases, obstruction of the air passage by phlegm or morbid changes due to invasion of pathogenic factors is common, which usually results in cough or asthma.

(2) Taking charge of the skin and hair. Here the "skin and hair" signify the entire body surface, which provides a superficial defense against external pathogenic factors. The body surface receives vital energy (*qi*) from the lungs. This energy is called "defensive energy" or "defensive *qi*." When the function of the lungs is diminished, the defensive energy becomes insufficient and the superficial resistance unsound, making one vulnerable to an attack by exogenous pathogenic factors, especially abnormal weather changes and certain epidemic pathogens. An invasion of the superficial part of the body by exogenous pathogenic factors usually has symptoms of the lungs (particularly upper respiratory symptoms) as its early manifestations.

(3) Regulating water passages. The lungs also regulate the circulation of body fluids and water metabolism. The lungs' dispersing function turns a part of the body fluids into sweat, while the lungs' descending function continuously sends body fluids down to the kidneys to be excreted as urine. The latter function is known as regulating water passages. If this function is impaired, edema in the upper portion of the body will occur.

### 5. The kidneys

The gross anatomical description of the kidneys in traditional Chinese medicine accords with that of Western medicine, though the former includes the suprarenal gland as a part of the kidneys. However, the functions of the kidneys in traditional Chinese medicine go far beyond the secretion of urine; many other important functions, such as reproduction, growth and development, are all attributed to this visceral organ. Thus, the kidneys are the foundation of the native or inborn constitution. Its main physiological functions can be summarized as follows:

(1) Storing essence and dominating reproduction, growth and development. The essence in the kidneys consists of two parts: the congenital essence inherited from the parents and the acquired essence derived from food. The former is essential for human

reproduction; the Chinese character 精 signifies both essence and semen. Congenital essence and acquired essence are interdependent. The parents' reproductive essences after fusion becomes the congenital essence of the embryo. After birth, the essence derived from food continuously nourishes the congenital essence. Both constitute the vital essence of the kidneys, making possible the child's growth and development. According to the *Canon of Medicine*, females at age 14 will begin menstrating and males at age 16 will begin having seminal emissions, both events signifying the onset of reproductive power. In other words, the vital essence of the kidneys transforms into reproductive essence which in turn becomes the congenital essence of the offspring. In this sense, "the kidneys" refers to the reproductive system, including the relevant endocrine glands. Thus, various sexual disorders and sterility or infertility are usually attributed to dysfunction or hypofunction of the kidneys and are effectively treated with kidney tonics.

(2) Producing marrow, dominating the bones and replenishing the brain. Marrow, including bone marrow and spinal marrow, is produced from the essence stored in the kidneys. Bone marrow in turn fills and nourishes the bones, so the bones' condition is closely related to the function of the kidneys. Deficiency of kidney essence is a common cause of defective skeletal development in children and other disorders of the bones which involve reduction of their solidity.

The upper part of the spinal cord connects with the brain, which is also called "the reservoir of marrow or medulla." Thus, some of the brain's functions, such as intelligence and nimbleness, are controlled by the kidneys.

(3) Dominating water metabolism. When the fluid sent down by the descending function of the lungs reaches the kidneys, it is speparated into two parts: the clear and the turbid. The clear fluid (the useful part) is retained, while the turbid fluid (the waste part) flows into the urinary bladder and is excreted as urine. According to traditional Chinese medical theory, the micturition function of the urinary bladder can only be accomplished with the assistance of the kidneys. Thus, "the kidneys" refers to the whole urinary system rather than just the two organic bodies located in the lumbar region.

(4) Helping taking in air. The kidneys help the lungs with inhalation. If this function is impaired, dyspnea or asthma may occur, characterized by breathing with prolonged exhalation and shortened inhalation.

### 6. The pericardium

The pericardium, the membrane surrounding the heart, is not generally regarded an independent organ. When exogenous pathogenic factors invade the heart, however, they usually encroach on the pericardium first. In fact, pericardium trouble is synonymous with heart trouble. In acupuncture, the Pericardium Meridian is as important as the Heart Meridian, and there is remarkable similarity in indications between the two meridians.

## II. The Fu organs

### 1. The small intestine

The small intestine receives food that has been partially digested in the stomach, further digests it, separates the essential from the waste, absorbs the useful substances and transfers the residues to the large intestine. Although the small intestine is important for digesting food and absorbing nutrients, digestive disorders are seldom diagnosed in terms of the small intestine. They are usually associated with the spleen, since the latter dominates the process of digestion and absorption as a part of transforming food and transporting food essence. Nevertheless, since fluids are also a part of the useful substance absorbed by the small intestine, abnormalities of the urine are sometimes attributed to this portion of the food canal.

### 2. The gallbladder

The gallbladder is attached to the liver. It stores bile and excretes it into the intestines to help digestion. Since bile is bitter and yellow, diseases of the gallbladder are usually manifested by bitterness in the mouth, vomit of bitter fluid, and yellow discoloration of the skin and sclera accompanied by digestive disorders. Traditional Chinese medicine also relates the gallbladder function to several mental activities, especially courage and the power of decision. Mental disorder characterized by susceptibility to fright, insomnia and dreamfulness is an example of a syndrome of the gallbladder. This medical theory is embodied in the Chinese language: "A man with a small gallbladder" is a coward.

### 3. The stomach

The stomach receives and temporarily stores food, partially digests it and transforms it into chyme, and then sends this downward to the small intestine. Therefore, the normal function of the stomach has a descending property. If the action of the stomach is in the reverse direction, nausea, vomiting, belching or regurgitation occurs.

### 4. The large intestine

The large intestine passes on the waste material sent down from the small intestine, absorbs part of the fluids and finally excretes the waste as feces. Disturbance of the large intestine usually gives rise to diarrhea or constipation.

### 5. The urinary bladder

The urinary bladder is a reservoir for urine, temporarily storing it and then eventually excreting it from the body. The urinary bladder's function is accomplished with the assistance of the kidneys. Problems with urination, such as enuresis or incontinence of urine, though ascribed to the urinary bladder, are also attributed to the kidneys.

### 6. *Sanjiao* (Triple Energizer)

*Sanjiao* is translated literally as triple energizer or triple heater, but its transliteration is also often used. *Sanjiao* is not a substantial organ, rather it is a functional system or a generalization of some of the functions of the *zang-fu* organs located in different sections of the body cavity. In this sense, *sanjiao*, or the triple energizer, refers to "the three portions of the body cavity." The *Canon of Medicine* summarizes the functions of the triple energizer in these figures of speech:

"The upper-*jiao* (or the thoracic cavity) is like a sprayer," because the heart and lungs housed there spread *qi* and blood throughout the body and send fluids down to the kidneys.

"The middle-*jiao* (or the upper abdominal cavity) resembles a fermentation vat," because the stomach and the spleen housed there decompose and digest food.

"The lower-*jiao* (or the lower abdominal cavity) works like rain gutters," because the kidneys, urinary bladder and large intestine housed there filter and drain off waste and surplus water.

# CHAPTER III    MATERIAL BASIS OF THE VITAL ACTIVITIES OF THE HUMAN BODY

*Qi*, blood, vital essence, body fluids and nutrients are fundamental substances. The *zang-fu* organs and all of the other organs and tissues of the human body depend on them in order to function.

## *QI* (VITAL ENERGY)

The concept of *qi* is based on an ancient, naive understanding of natural phenomena. In this concept, *qi* is the basic element which constitutes the cosmos and produces everything in the world through its movements and changes. In medicine, *qi* has two meanings: It is the basic substance that maintains the activities of human life, and it is the motive force or energy required for life's activities. *Qi*, either as basic element or energy, is invisible; what can be perceived are the functional activities *qi* promotes. For example, *qi* of the kidneys implies the functional activities of the kidneys, and *qi*-deficiency of the kidneys actually means hypofunction of the kidneys.

*Qi* consists of the inborn and the acquired. Inborn *qi* originates from the innate essence stored in the kidneys which has been inherited from the parents. Acquired *qi* is formed by combining the food essence obtained through digestion and oxygen inhaled through the lungs. Together, inborn and acquired *qi* constitute genuine *qi* (or vital energy), which circulates in the body, is distributed to each organ and tissue and is responsible for all the body's functional activities and its resistance to disease.

The meridians and collaterals form the passageways through which *qi* circulates. They traverse the human body, linking the internal organs with each other and with the various tissues and organs located elsewhere. With its view of the body as an organic, integrated whole, traditional Chinese medicine emphasizes the dynamic force of *qi* in uniting the body's organs and tissues.

## BLOOD

Blood circulates through the vessels together with nutrients. The essence of food, derived from digestion and absorption, combines with fluids containing nutrients to form blood. The kidneys also contribute to forming blood because they store essence that produces bone marrow. Furthermore, there is a reciprocal relationship between essence and blood, i.e., essence can be transformed into blood, and vice versa. Thus, blood production depends upon the functional activities of various visceral organs, including the stomach, spleen, heart and kidneys, as well as these ingredients — essence, nutrients, *qi* and bone marrow.

The heart, with the help of the lungs, promotes blood circulation. The spleen keeps the blood flowing within the vessels. The liver stores blood, serving as a reservoir to regulate the volume of circulating blood.

## VITAL ESSENCE

As discussed in the previous chapter, essence has two meanings just as *qi* has. Congenital essence is closely related to reproduction, and is also called reproductive essence. Acquired essence is produced from the nutrients derived from food and is distributed to all the tissues and organs of the body. The former is the origin of the human life, and the latter is the material basis of the body's activities. Without the former the body could not exist, and hence there would be no acquired essence. However, acquired essence should constantly nourish congenital essence. That is why insufficiency of acquired essence may lead to sexual disturbances and sterility or infertility. Although essence and semen share the same character in Chinese, the reproductive essence in traditional medicine is by no means confined to males.

All *zang* organs have their own vital essence. When essence is abundant in these organs, part of the essence will be stored in the kidneys. When the organs need more essence, the kidneys supply it. Furthermore, the acquired essence stored in the kidneys can be transformed into reproductive essence after adolescence. Therefore, in traditional Chinese medicine, sexual overindulgence can cause disease because it not only consumes kidney essence but also impairs other *zang* organs.

The vital essence is the material basis of all life and throughout life it is incessantly consumed and at the same time constantly replenished. Not only is it responsible for reproduction, it is closely related with the process of growth, development and aging. Senility results when vital essence declines.

## BODY FLUIDS

Body fluids come from food and drink, and exist in the blood and the interstices of tissues. The *Canon of Medicine* includes a brief description of the complicated process of forming, distributing and excreting body fluids, i.e., water metabolism:

> After drink enters the stomach, it is absorbed and transmitted to the spleen. The spleen sends the essential fluids to the lungs, which, in turn, regulate water passages, sending the fluid downward until it is introduced into the urinary bladder. Thus, the essential fluids are distributed throughout the body and flow in all the vessels and channels of the organs and tissues.

Present day traditional Chinese medicine describes the formation, distribution and excretion of body fluids as follows: Having entered the stomach, food and drink are partially digested and sent to the small intestine and then the large intestine. In the intestines the essential fluid is absorbed and then transported by the spleen to the heart and lungs. The residue of food, which normally contains a small amount of water, is excreted as feces. The essential fluid is dispersed from the heart and lungs throughout the body to nourish various organs and tissues. The fluid that comes to the skin may be excreted as sweat. By their descending function, the lungs regulate water passages and send some body fluids down to the kidneys and on to the urinary bladder to be excreted as urine.

Pathogenic heat disrupts this process and consumes body fluids, as do the following factors: (1) insufficient fluid intake; (2) dysfunction of the stomach in receiving food and drink, e.g., vomiting; (3) dysfunction of the stomach in sending down the fluid, as seen in pylorus stenosis; (4) diseases of the intestines, with diarrhea causing profuse loss of fluid in fecal discharges; (5) dysfunction of the kidneys, with polyuria as seen in diabetes; and (6) excessive sweating, e.g., due to improper administration of diaphoretics.

# MUTUAL RELATIONS AMONG *QI,* BLOOD, VITAL ESSENCE AND BODY FLUIDS.

## I. Relation between *qi* and blood

According to the *Canon of Medicine,* "*Qi* is the dynamic force of the blood flow, while blood is the material base of *qi*." Clinically, deficiency of *qi* often leads to deficiency of blood, and deficiency of blood, in turn, frequently results in deficiency of *qi*. For instance, deficiency of *qi* of the spleen may give rise to anemia due to diminished absorption of nutrients. In this case blood tonics are not sufficient to treat the anemia, satisfactory therapeutic results can only be obtained when drugs that replenish *qi* are added.

A close relationship also exists between the circulation of *qi* and blood. Stagnation of the flow of *qi* often causes blood stasis, and blood stasis, in turn, usually aggravates the stagnation of *qi*. For instance, patients suffering from hepatitis usually complain of distending pain over the hepatic area (stagnation of *qi* in the liver), but as the disease advances hepatomegaly accompanied by stabbing pain (stasis of blood in the liver) will occur. Furthermore, as blood is kept in circulation by *qi*, deficiency of *qi* may lead to blood stasis. For example, congestive heart failure involves blood stasis due to deficiency of *qi* of the heart.

In addition, the spleen controls blood, i.e., it keeps the blood circulating within the vessels. This function also depends upon the action of *qi*. If the spleen lacks *qi*, derangement of blood circulation, manifested as chronic hemorrhagic disorders, may occur.

## II. Relation between *qi* and body fluids

The formation, distribution and excretion of body fluids depend upon the action of *qi*. Insufficient function of the spleen and the kidneys is one of the factors in the pathogenesis of edema. In other words, deficiency of *qi* of the spleen and the kidneys may cause derangement of water circulation and excretion, and lead to excessive retention of water in the body. On the other hand, excessive accumulation of fluids in the body, in turn, impedes the normal circulation of *qi*, so that in a severely edematous patient anorexia, abdominal distension and even nausea and vomiting occur, indicating deranged flow of *qi* in the spleen and the stomach. Furthermore, excessive loss of body fluids due to excessive perspiration, repeated vomiting or severe diarrhea may lead to prostration of *qi*.

## III. Relation between blood and vital essence

Blood and vital essence are of the same origin. Both are derived from food nutrients. Clinically, deficiency of vital essence is apt to cause deficiency of blood, and deficiency of blood is often accompanied by deficiency of vital essence.

## IV. Relation between blood and body fluids

Fluids are an important constituent of blood, and turn into interstitial fluids when they are extravasated. Massive bleeding usually leads to deficiency of body fluids, bringing on symptoms such as thirst and oliguria. On the other hand, deficiency of body fluids may cause condensation of blood. That is why diaphoretics ordinarily used in treating exterior syndromes are contraindicated in patients with hemorrhage even though there is an exterior syndrome present.

# CHAPTER IV   ETIOLOGY AND PATHOGENESIS

Any system of medicine must answer the questions What is health and What is disease? Traditional Chinese medicine holds that health exists when *yin* and *yang* within the human body and between the human body and the external environment are kept in a normal, dynamic balance. If the balance is impaired, disease will result. Therefore, an imbalance of *yin-yang* is always considered the general pathogenesis of disease.

Pathogenic factors impair the normal *yin-yang* balance. They may originate in the external environment or within the human body. In any disease pathogenic factors attack the body, while on the other hand the vital energy resists them. Disease is the struggle of the vital energy against the pathogenic factors.

Many statements in the *Canon of Medicine* relate to the battle between the vital energy and the pathogenic factors, emphasizing the resisting capacity of the former against the latter: "When there is abundant vital energy in the body, invasion of the pathogenic factors is impossible." "When the pathogenic factor enters the body, the vital energy is bound to be insufficient." "A pathogenic factor, such as wind, rain, cold or heat, itself is unable to cause damage to the human body unless there is insufficiency of the vital energy. Some people with good resistance, though caught in a heavy rain and strong wind, do not get ill. Therefore, merely the pathogenic factor itself is not enough to cause a disease."

The limitations of natural science and technology during ancient times prevented traditional Chinese medicine practitioners from discovering pathogens, such as bacteria and viruses. Practitioners did discover etiological factors by observing and analyzing clinical manifestations. Though not entirely logical from the modern point of view, this etiology is very useful in clinical practice since it is closely related to therapeutic effects.

Pathogenic factors are usually classified into two groups: the exogenous, which cause exogenous diseases or external infections, and the endogenous, which cause endogenous diseases or internal injuries. Exogenous pathogenic factors include abnormal atmospheric changes, pestilential pathogens, trauma, etc. Common endogenous pathogenic factors are emotions (such as joy, anger, melancholy, anxiety, grief, fear and fright), improper diet, overfatigue, overindulgence in sex, etc.

Among exogenous pathogenic factors, abnormal atmospheric changes are most significant. Not only do they cause seasonal diseases, such as colds in winter and heatstroke in summer, they also cause most infectious diseases marked by seasonal epidemicity.

There are six kinds of atmospheric changes: wind, cold, summer-heat, damp, dryness and fire (intense heat). In a narrow sense, these factors are closely related to changes in the weather. If the weather suddenly becomes too hot or too cold it changes out of season, such as a warm spell in winter or a cold snap in summer, it can become pathogenic because the body is unable to adopt to these changes. Of course, there is no clear-cut line between normal and abnormal or nonpathogenic and pathogenic. A sudden violent change may not harm individuals with a strong constitution, while those with a weak constitution may find even a mild change pathogenic. Therefore, a practitioner cannot determine the cause of a disease merely by observing atmospheric changes.

Determining pathogenic atmospheric factors depends chiefly upon observing clinical manifestations rather than searching for the pathogenic factors themselves. For example, if the diagnosis is "invasion by wind," this does not necessarily mean that the patient has been in a draught. It merely means that the clinical manifestations indicate the characteristic features of the natural wind.

Furthermore, clinical manifestations resembling the properties of natural wind may not be caused by exogenic factors; they may be the result of an attack by endogenic factors. Therefore, the pathogenic factors of wind, cold, heat, damp, dryness and fire may originate from outside through abnormal atmospheric changes and pathogens which cause infectious diseases or from inside through pathogenic factors produced within the body by other causes.

### 1. Wind and wind syndromes

Wind is air in motion. Symptoms with the following characteristics are caused by the wind and grouped under the heading wind syndromes:

(1) Symptoms or diseases with sudden onset and quick disappearance, e.g., urticaria and angioneuro-edema.

(2) Diseases with lesions that move from one place to to another, e.g., rheumatic arthritis with migratory joint pain.

(3) General diseases with marked symptoms in the head and face, e.g., acute nephritis with puffy eyelids.

(4) Symptoms or diseases characterized by sudden onset of abnormal involuntary movements or sensation of abnormal movements, e.g., tremors, twitching, convulsions, vertigo, fainting and apoplexy.

(5) Aversion to wind and sweating (as if the wind blew the pores open), as seen in certain patterns of colds and in patients with deficiency of vital energy.

Thus, wind syndromes can be classified into two cateories: exogenous wind syndromes (such as colds and acute rheumatic arthritis after exposure to wind and cold) and endogenous wind syndromes (such as vertigo and stroke). However, one cannot determine causation merely on the basis of similarities in clinical manifestations. This kind of "aetiological" classification is actually based upon therapeutic effects. For instance, colds ("catching wind"), urticaria ("wind rash"), rheumatic arthritis with migratory pain ("windy arthritis") and acute nephritis at the onset ("windy edema') can all be treated with wind-dispelling drugs, such as *Herb Schizonepetae, Radix Ledebouriellae* and *Herba Ephedrae*. Endogenous wind syndromes, whether they occur in hypertension, Meniere's syndrome or cerebrovascular accidents, can be treated with drugs to subdue the endogenous wind (sedatives and anticonvulsives).

### 2. Cold and cold syndromes

Cold is an important pathogenic factor commonly seen in clinical practice. It can be of exogenous origin (exposure to cold) and endogenous origin (decreased heat metabolism). Syndromes caused by cold have the following characteristics:

(1) Cold consumes heat energy of the body, resulting in chilliness with cold limbs.

(2) Cold causes contraction of the muscles.

(3) Cold causes stagnation of *qi* and blood manifested by pain. (Pain caused by cold is characterized by its severity, fixed location and exaggerated harshness during and after exposure to cold.)

(4) Cold often attacks the gastro-intestinal tract causing abdominal pain, vomiting and diarrhea.

A key way to differentiate exogenous from endogenous cold syndromes is by their response to heat. The chilliness of an exogenous cold syndrome, particularly if it occurs as an early symptom of an infectious disease, cannot be alleviated by heavy clothing and a warm environment. On the other hand, the chilliness due to decreased heat metabolism in endogenous cold syndromes can be easily alleviated by applying warmth.

### 3. Damp and damp syndromes

A damp atmosphere and wet environments may cause disease, but not all damp syndromes are due to exogneous damp. In many cases, dysfunction of the visceral organs, especially the spleen, produces damp within the body. The characteristics of damp syndromes are as follows:

(1) Damp makes things sticky, thus diseases caused by damp often linger.

(2) Damp makes things heavy, thus the patient suffering from damp feels heaviness in the head (as if the head were tightly bound) and in the body and limbs.

(3) Damp can turn into turbid liquid, thus turbid discharges (such as morbid leucorrhea, turbid urine and exudation from skin lesions) are usually attributed to pathogenic damp.

(4) Damp may impede the normal flow of *qi*, thus a sensation of fullness in the chest, dyspnea and cough with profuse expectoration may occur when the function of the lungs is impaired; epigastric or abdominal distension, anorexia, nausea, vomiting and diarrhea may occur when the function of the spleen and stomach is involved.

The onset of the disease and the location of pathological lesions help differentiate between exogenous and endogenous damp. Damp syndromes of acute onset especially after exposure to damp (e.g., being caught in a rain) with symptoms involving the body exterior (such as fever and chilliness, headache as if the head were tightly bound and pain, swelling and a heavy sensation in the joints) indicate an attack of exogenous damp. However, when the visceral organs are involved, the differentiation is more difficult. For example, in cases of exogenous damp, dysfunction of the spleen and stomach is the effect, damp the cause. In cases of endogenous damp, however, damp is a product of the disease, dysfunction of the spleen the cause.

### 4. Dryness and syndromes of dryness

Exogenous dryness frequently occurs in autumn because of the dry weather. Since the upper respiratory tract is directly exposed to the dry atmosphere, dryness can easily attack the lungs, with dry mouth, dry lips, dry nose, dry throat and dry cough as typical symptoms. However, factors other than the dry atmosphere can cause dryness in the body, namely, deficiency of body fluids, such as excessive administration of warming and dessicating drugs, profuse vomiting, severe diarrhea, excessive perspiration, massive haemorrhage, high fever and chronic consumption. These states of fluid deficiency belong to the syndrome of endogenous dryness which is clinically characterized by wizened skin, parched lips, dry cough, thirst and constipation. Differentiation between exogenous and endogenous dryness is usually easy since the primary factors of endogenous dryness are evident. Moreover, the symptoms caused by exogenous dryness are usually limited to the respiratory tract, while those caused by endogenous dryness occur throughout the body.

### 5. Heat and heat syndromes

Although high temperatures may cause disease, such as heatstroke, in most cases heat refers to pathogenic factors that induce fever, thirst, irritability, scanty concentrated urine, constipation, reddened tongue with yellow coating and rapid pulse, i.e., heat syndromes. Besides exogenous heat, other exogenous factors, such as wind, cold, damp and dryness, can be transformed into heat and cause heat syndromes.

Endogenous pathogenic factors, frequently due to deficiency of *yin*, can also produce heat syndromes. Techniques for differentiating syndromes caused by exogenous and endogenous heat will be discussed elsewhere.

### 6. Fire and fire syndromes

Traditional Chinese medicine attributes acute inflammations with local redness and heat or fever to fire. Fire or intense heat can impair body fluids, leading to dryness in the mouth, thirst and desire for drinks, constipation and oliguria. It can also injure the blood vessels, causing bleeding. Exogenous pathogenic factors can directly cause fire syndromes. Here, exogenous fire refers to any pathogen that can cause local inflammation. However, many other pathogenic factors, either exogenous or endogenous, may also turn into fire and produce fire syndromes. For example, emotional factors may cause functional derangement of the liver or the heart, causing a syndrome of liver-fire or heart-fire.

When endogenous factors are the genesis of fire syndromes, their underlying causes may be related to emotions, diet, stress or inactivity.

Emotional factors (joy, anger, melancholy, anxiety, grief, fear and fright) reflect one's mental state. They are physiological phenomena under normal conditions, but if they are in excess (either due to the intensity of the stimuli or the hypersensitivity of the individual to the stimuli), they may lead to disease. Here, the emotions, not the stimuli in the environment, are considered pathogenic factors which directly cause dysfunction of the *zang-fu* organs and disturb circulation of *qi* and blood. Thus, diseases caused by emotional factors are called endogenous diseases or internal injuries.

Various emotional changes selectively injure different *zang-fu* organs, e.g., anger injures the liver and anxiety injures the spleen. Clinically, disorders caused by emotional factors are most often seen in troubles of the heart, liver, spleen and stomach.

Diet can also cause fire syndromes. Improper food intake, including voracious eating, eating excessive amounts of raw or cold food, partiality for a particular food or intake of unsanitary food, may injure the stomach and the spleen.

Generally speaking, improper food intake causes digestive disorders. If the spleen and stomach are still functioning but become overloaded, indigestion of the excess type will occur. It should be treated with digestants and drugs to remove the undigested food retained in the stomach and intestines. However, if the spleen and stomach have already been impaired, digestive disorders may occur even when the patient is on a normal or light diet. In these cases, the practitioner should administer tonics to strengthen the function of the spleen and stomach.

Strain, fatigue and lack of physical exercise can also affect the *zang-fu* organs. Lack of necessary physical exertion may retard circulation of *qi* and blood, weaken the *zang-fu* organs and lower the body's resistance to disease. Prolonged strain consumes one's *qi* and blood, and can cause deficiency syndromes. Traditional Chinese medicine also emphasizes the adverse effects of sexual overindulgence. Because semen is part of the vital essence, and because the vital essence is stored in the kidneys, excessive sexual activity usually leads to deficiency of the kidneys and then deficiency of the energy derived from the essence.

Although endogenous pathogenic factors can cause diseases by directly injuring the *zang-fu* organs, the pathogenesis is usually complicated through intermediate links. For example, anger is apt to injure the liver, but "injury of the liver by anger" is seldom diagnosed alone. Anger usually impairs the normal flow of *qi* in the liver, causing stagnation of the liver-*qi*, which may in turn lead to blood stasis and then other secondary disturbances. Therefore, stagnation of *qi* and stasis of blood, though pathological products, may also act as pathogenic factors. Similar conditions occur when anxiety or improper diet cause dysfunction of the spleen, which in turn produces phlegm.

### 7. Stagnated *Qi* and syndrome of *Qi* stagnation

*Qi* is the motive force of various *zang-fu* functions, so stagnation of *qi* is by no means confined to the liver. Anger may cause stagnation of *qi* in the liver, but emotional factors can also stagnate *qi* in other *zang-fu* organs, such as the heart, the stomach and the spleen. Pain and distention are common manifestations of stagnated *qi*. Generally speaking, stagnated *qi* causes pain that is usually distending without fixed location, often moving from one place to another, and temporarily alleviated by discharge of gas, e.g., belching may relieve distending pain in the stomach.

### 8. Blood stasis and syndrome of blood stasis

"*Qi* is the dynamic force of blood flow," says the *Canon of Medicine*. Stagnated *qi* causes blood stasis, which in turn becomes a pathogenic factor that causes various disorders. Pain that is severe, stabbing in character and fixed in location is a common clinical feature of blood stasis.

The concept of blood stasis in traditional Chinese medicine is much broader than that in modern Western medicine. In the latter, blood stasis refers to retardation or stoppage of blood flow within the vessels, especially venous congestion. In traditonal Chinese medicine, the most typical case of blood stasis is extravasation, in which the extravasated blood stops flowing. Thus, the term blood stasis has several usages. First, in traumatology, blood stasis refers to lesions and wounds with ecchymosis. Second, when stagnated blood blocks the blood vessel, the circulating blood will escape through bleeding. Bleeding with discharge of dark blood and blood clots is usually attributed to blood stasis. Third, accumulation of stagnated blood may cause masses to form. Hence, hepato-splenomegaly and even some kinds of tumours are considered masses formed by blood stasis. Fourth, any condition accompanied by stabbing pain fixed in location and other signs, such as purple spots on the tongue or purplish tongue, is often due to blood stasis. Furthermore, blood congestion, thrombosis formation and vascular ischemia can be all classified as due to blood stasis.

### 9. Phlegm and the syndrome of phlegm

Functional disorders of the lungs, spleen and kidneys may cause retention of excessive fluids in the body. If a large amount of excessive water accumulates subcutaneously, edema occurs. If the excessive fluid accumulates in a certain part of the body and condenses, phlegm is formed.

Phlegm affecting the lungs causes cough, asthma and expectoration of sputum. Phlegm misting the heart (mind) causes loss of consciousness in apoplexy. Phlegm combined with fire disturbing the normal function of the heart causes epilepsy, hysteria and mania. Phlegm blocking the meridians and collaterals causes numbness of limbs in mild cases, and hemiplegia in serious conditions. Phlegm retained subcutaneously becomes masses or nodules, such as enlarged lymph nodes.

Why are these various pathological conditions attributed to phlegm and grouped together under the category of phlegm syndrome? The ancient texts give many answers, but the most convincing one is that the practitioner can effectively treat all these conditions using the method called "to dispel phlegm."

# CHAPTER V   THE GENERAL PARAMETERS OF SYNDROME DIAGNOSIS

In traditional Chinese medicine the diagnosis of the syndrome is more important than the diagnosis of the disease. The syndrome or symptom-complex is not merely a collection of symptoms and signs, it comprises the following components: location of the pathological changes, cause and pathogenensis of the disease, nature of the syndrome and the ability of the body to resist the pathogenic factors. The general parameters for differentiating syndromes can be summarized into exterior versus interior, cold versus heat and deficiency versus excess.

## EXTERIOR VERSUS INTERIOR

Exterior and interior relate to the depth or location of the disease, with exterior being the superficial portion of the body, including the subcutaneous tissue, sweat glands, skeletal muscles and the meridians and collaterals running through this portion, and interior being the visceral organs (*zang-fu*).

Invading exogenous pathogenic factors (exogenous affections) usually cause diseases of the exterior. Their common clinical manifestations are: chilliness and fever, headache, aching of the body or joints, thin coating of the tongue and floating or superficial pulse. Exterior syndromes may also involve upper respiratory symptoms, such as stuffy nose, sore throat and cough.

Interior syndromes, associated with diseases of the visceral organs, may be caused in any of the following three ways:

1. Transmission of exogenous pathogenic factors from the exterior to the interior. For instance, following an exterior syndrome with chills, fever, headache and floating pulse, a high fever without chills and accompanied by dyspnea, expectoration of yellow sticky sputum, chest pain, dire thirst, reddened tongue with thick yellow coating and forceful and rapid pulse may occur. These symptoms would indicate an interior syndrome caused by the transmission of the pathogenic factor from the exterior to the interior — i.e., a syndrome of heat in the lungs transmitted from the exterior.

2. Direct attack of exogenous pathogenic factors on the visceral organs. For example, catching a cold may result in vomiting, abdominal pain, diarrhea and borborygmi, indicating that the stomach and intestines had been affected — i.e., a syndrome of direct attack of the interior by cold.

3. Dysfunctioning of the visceral organs due to internal injuries. For instance, after an emotional turmoil, headache, dizziness, bloodshot eyes and tinnitus with taut rapid pulse and reddened tongue and yellow coating may occur, indicating hyperactivity of the liver — i.e., a syndrome of fire in the liver.

Differentiating exterior from interior syndromes involves several key points. Exogenous pathogenic factors cause most exterior syndromes. Exterior syndromes occur at the early stage of exogenous affections and last for a short period of time. As a rule, manifestations include chills or aversion to cold (or wind), thin coating of the tongue and floating pulse. Among these, presence of chills and aversion to cold (or wind) are of crucial importance. Dysfunction of the visceral organs characterize interior syndromes. If there is fever, chills and aversion to cold (or wind) do not accompany it. The other symptoms of interior sydromes are as diverse as the visceral organs with which they are associated.

In addition to those mentioned above, two other general syndromes relate to the exterior and interior. One involves an affection located between the exterior and the interior, marked by alternate fever and chills, a feeling of fullness or pain in the chest and costal regions, a bitter taste in the mouth, dry throat, nausea, loss of appetite and taut pulse. The other concerns an affection of both the exterior and the interior, marked by simultaneous exterior and interior symptom complexes.

## COLD VERSUS HEAT

Differentiating between the cold or heat nature of a syndrome is important because it provides the basis for administering drugs that are hot or cold in property.*

Syndromes caused by pathogenic heat, summer heat or dryness are mostly of a heat nature, while those caused by pathogenic cold at the early stage of the disease are often of a cold nature. Moreover, deficiency of *yin* and *yang* may also lead to heat and cold syndromes, respectively. In combination with the depth of the disease (i.e., the exterior and interior) cold and heat syndromes can be divided into four categories: cold in the exterior, heat in the exterior, cold in the interior and heat in the interior.

The exterior cold syndrome has marked chilliness and mild fever, no sweat, thin white tongue coating and floating and tense pulse as its symptoms.

Fever with mild chilliness or intolerance of wind characterize the exterior heat syndrome. This syndrome may also involve mild sweating and a little thirst. The tongue coating will be thin, but may be somewhat yellowish, and the pulse will be floating and rapid.

Cold and heat syndromes of the interior are much more complicated.

In cold and heat syndromes, different causes lead to different manifestations. Also, the interior of the body includes many visceral organs, each with its own physiological functions which if diseased, display different clinical manifestations. Generally speaking, the cold syndrome of a visceral organ refers to its hypofunction, heat syndrome to its hyperfunction.

Even with this great variety in mainfestations, cold and heat syndromes each have a set of characteristic features. Pallor, intolerance of cold, absence of thirst, loose stools, clear profuse urine, pale tongue with white coating and slow pulse characterize interior cold syndromes. If there is pain, it is aggravated by cold and alleviated by warmth. If

---

* All herbal drugs fall under two general categories, i.e., cold and cool versus hot and warm. For cold syndromes, drugs warm or hot in property should be used, while for heat syndromes, drugs cool or cold in property are indicated.

there is expectoration, the sputum is thin, frothy and whitish. On the contrary, flushed face, fever or feverishness, thirst, irritability and restlessness, constipation, deep-colored scanty urine, reddened tongue with yellow coating and rapid pulse characterize interior heat syndromes. If there is pain, it is aggravated by heat and alleviatd by cold. If there is expectoration, the sputum is thick, sticky and yellowish.

While these criteria help physicians distinguish between cold and heat syndromes in most cases, special attention should be paid to the following aspects:

1. Transformation of cold into heat and vice versa. It is common for exogenous cold to transform into heat after penetrating the interior of the body. The exterior cold syndrome begins with chills, stuffy nose, headache and general aching, thin white coating of the tongue and floating tense pulse. Later, a high fever develops and the chills disappear, the tongue becomes reddened and its coating turns thick and yellow and the pulse becomes rapid. Thus, the transformation from exterior cold syndrome to interior heat syndrome is complete.

2. Coexistence and interlocking of cold and heat. Jumbled cases, in which cold and heat syndromes coexist, have four main patterns: (1) cold in the exterior and heat in the interior; (2) heat in the exterior and cold in the interior; (3) cold in the upper part of the body and heat in the lower part; and (4) heat in the upper part of the body and cold in the lower part. For example, exogenous pathogenic cold may transform into heat after penetrating into the interior of the body, yet the cold in the exterior is still present. Both syndromes coexist. The patient may have chills, headache and be unable to sweat, and at the same time have fever with irritability, thirst and constipation.

3. Pseudo-cold and pseudo-heat. Symptoms of pseudo-cold or pseudo-heat are often misleading and require careful identification. If the patient feels chilly but doesn't want to be thickly covered, if the limbs feel cold, but the chest and abdomen feel hot, the patient is experiencing a heat syndrome, even though these symytoms appear to be cold in nature. If the patient feels hot yet wishes to be thickly covered, feels thirsty but drinks little, moves restlessly while being mentally quiescent, has a tongue coating that is black but moistened, the patient is suffering from a cold syndrome, since these manifestations are really pseudo-heat symptoms.

## DEFICIENCY VERSUS EXCESS

Deficiency and excess define opposing forces — the pathogenic factors which attack the body and the body's antipathogenic factors which resist them. Deficiency refers to a deficiency in the body's resistance; excess refers to an excess of pathogenic factors. When pathogenic factors are low and body resistance high, the body is in a healthy state.

There are three broad categories of syndromes related to deficiency and excess: (1) deficiency syndromes, which are manifested as insufficient body resistance and minimal influence from pathogenic factors; (2) excess syndromes, which are characterized by a fierce struggle between strong pathogenic factors and a body that is equally strong in resisting them; and (3) complicated syndromes of deficiency and excess, which are characterized by weakened body resistance which fails to contend with the pathogenic factor while it is active. Complicated syndromes can be further divided into two types:

syndromes of deficiency complicated with excess and syndromes of excess complicated with deficiency.

Traditional Chinese medicine classifies deficiency syndromes based on the body function which is deficient, such as deficiency of *yin* (vital essence) of the heart, insufficiency of *yang* (vital function) of the kidneys and weakness of *qi* (vital energy) of the spleen. Excess syndromes break down according to the categories of pathogenic factors and the consequent response of the body or viscera, such as accumulation of heat in the stomach, invasion of the spleen by cold-damp and flaming up of liver fire.

Deficiency and excess syndromes have many manifestations. Spontaneous sweating, pale tongue and floating and relaxed pulse characterize the exterior syndrome of deficiency type, or exterior deficiency syndrome. An exterior syndrome of excess type, or exterior excess syndrome, refers to an exterior cold syndrome characterized by chilliness, thin white tongue coating, floating and tense pulse and no sweating. Thus, the chief criterion for differentiating between deficiency and excess types in exterior syndromes is the presence or absence of sweating accompanying the chills.

In interior syndromes, the conditions are much more complicated. Generally speaking, an interior syndrome of deficiency type, or interior deficiency syndrome, usually appears in a long-standing disease. In addition to various symptoms due to the involvement of the *zang-fu* organs, the symptoms of an interior deficiency syndrome are weakness or emaciation, lassitude, shortness of breath, spontaneous or night sweating, pain alleviated by pressure, no tongue coating or thin coating and thready or feeble pulse.

Interior syndrome of excess type, or interior excess syndrome, is usually seen in a recent disease. Its clinical manifestations vary with the *zang-fu* organ involved and will be discussed in Chapter VI. If there is pain, it is aggravated by pressure or accompanied by tenderness. The tongue coating is usually thick or greasy, and the pulse forceful.

The nature of the disease, i.e., cold and heat, provides another subcategory of interior excess and deficiency syndromes. Interior cold syndromes of excess type are not common in clinical practice. Exogenous cold directly attacking the stomach and intestines is one example. Most cases of interior cold syndrome are of the deficiency type, particularly related to deficiency of *yang*.

Interior heat syndrome of excess type is common, not only in febrile diseases due to exogenous affections but also in diseases due to internal injuries without fever. In cases of febrile disease, the syndrome is characterized by high fever, flushed face, thirst, preference for cold drink, constipation, red tongue with yellow coating and rapid and forceful pulse. In cases of internal injuries, the clinical manifestations of the syndrome are diversified and related to the involvement of the *zang-fu* organs. For instance, a fit of anger may cause a sudden attack of dizziness and tinnitus accompanied by flushed face, burning pain in the hypochondriac regions, dryness and bitterness in the mouth, reddened tongue with yellow coating and taut rapid pulse. This would indicate a syndrome of excessive liver fire, an interior heat syndrome of excess type.

Interior heat and cold syndromes of deficiency type are often associated with deficiency of *yin* and *yang*, respectively. Deficiency of *yin* may bring on an interior heat syndrome of deficiency type. This condition has afternoon fever, malar flush, dry mouth and throat, feverish sensation in palms and soles, night sweating, constipation, concentrated urine, reddened tongue without coating or with little coating and thready and rapid pulse as its manifestations.

Deficiency of *yang* usually gives rise to an interior cold syndrome of deficiency type. Its clinical manifestations are chillness, cold limbs, pallor, absence of thirst, spontaneous sweating, loose stools, dilute urine, pale tongue with white coating and feeble and slow pulse.

Syndromes of deficiency and excess may also coexist and are frequently seen in clinical practice. Broadly speaking, when endogenous pathogenic factors are secondary to insufficient visceral functions as the cause of a condition, the condition is a syndrome of deficiency complicated with excess. When exogenous pathogenic factors cause consumption of vital energy, essence or visceral functions, the condition is a syndrome of excess complicated by deficiency. For instance, according to traditional Chinese medicine, chronic nephritis with nephrotic syndrome is considered a hypofunction of the spleen and the kidneys with water-damp in flood. It is a deficiency syndrome because the formation of water-damp is due to the hypofunction of the spleen and the kidneys, but it is also complicated by an excess of water-damp.

In summary, exterior versus interior, cold versus heat, and deficiency versus excess are general parameters to use in analyzing diseased conditions. Though clinical manifestations and pathological changes may be very complex, these parameters provide the basis for accurate diagnosis.

# CHAPTER VI  DIAGNOSIS AND TREATMENT ACCORDING TO THE PATHOLOGICAL CHANGES OF VISCERA (*ZANG-FU*)

Of the several ways to diagnose syndromes, diagnosing pathological changes of the viscera (*zang-fu*) is the most useful. This book describes this method in detail. Using this method along with the general parameters described in Chapter V will result in accurate diagnoses of the diseases of internal medicine.

## Section I  SYNDROMES OF THE LIVER AND THE GALLBLADDER

The liver is located in the right hypochondriac region, but its meridian branches into the bilateral costal and hypochondriac regions. The liver stores blood, smoothes and regulates the flow of *qi* and blood and controls the tendons. The gallbladder is attached to the liver. It stores bile. Since these two organs are related, diseases of the gallbladder are often considered from the view of the liver.

## SYMPTOMS AND SIGNS

### I. Symptoms and signs due to insufficient storage of blood in the liver

The *Canon of Medicine* describes the blood-storing function of the liver thus: "One can see with his eyes, walk with his feet, grasp with his hands and hold with his fingers only when the eyes, feet, hands and fingers are supplied with blood by the liver; when one goes to bed at night, a part of the circulating blood returns to the liver." In other words, physical activity (movements of the joints and limbs are considered the function of the tendons) and vision need blood supplied by the liver. If the blood stored in the liver is insufficient, pallor, blurring of the vision and dryness of the eyes, spasms of the tendons and muscles, numbness of the limbs and scanty menstrual flow with a prolonged cycle in women will occur. In addition, there may be massive bleeding, such as hematemesis or massive uterine bleeding, when liver fire (e.g., after a fit of anger) impairs the liver's ability to store blood.

### II. Symptoms and signs due to impaired smoothing and regulating of *qi* and blood

Smoothing and regulating *qi* involves several aspects: keeping oneself in a calm and merry mood, maintaining the smooth flow of *qi* along the Liver Meridian, regulating the flow of bile and regulating the functions of the spleen and the stomach. If the function of smoothing and regulating *qi* is impaired, stagnation of *qi* occurs, marked by irritability, irascibility, distension and pain in the regions where the Liver Meridian traverses (such as the hypochondriac, mammary, pectoral, lateral abdominal and inguinal regions), digestive disorders (such as anorexia, belching, vomiting, abdominal distension or diarrhea) and in some cases jaundice.

Because *qi* is the force behind blood circulation, serious stagnation of *qi* for a considerable length of time will cause blood stasis, resulting in pricking pain fixed in location and the formation of masses, such as hepatosplenomegaly or gynecological tumour.

Excessive or persistent stagnation of the liver *qi* will turn into liver fire, manifested by headache, dizziness, marked irascibility, tinnitus, impairment of hearing and blood-shot eyes. The liver fire can, in turn, become wind. The common manifestations of liver wind are vertigo, tremors and convulsions.

## III. Symptoms and signs due to dysfunction of the gallbladder

The common manifestations of gall bladder diseases are pain in the right hypochondriac region (where the gall bladder is situated), bitterness in the mouth, vomiting of bitter fluid (because of the bitter taste of the bile) and jaundice (due to accumulation of bile in the body). These symptoms are discussed in greater detail below.

1. Headache. Headache is a common symptom seen in liver disorders with exuberant liver *yang*, either of excess type (liver fire) or of deficiency type (exuberance of *yang* secondary to deficiency of liver *yin*). It is often accompanied by dizziness, fidgets and irascibility and precipitated or aggravated by an emotional upset. Of course, headaches are by no means confined to liver disorders. They are more frequently a symptom of exogenous affections, particularly affection by wind.

2. Dizziness. The most common cause of dizziness is exuberance of liver *yang*. Dizziness may also be due to an insufficient supply of *qi*, blood or vital essence to the brain, or phlegm interfering with the brain. Dizziness due to exuberance of the liver *yang* may be either of excess or deficiency type. The former is characterized by an acute onset and is accompanied by other manifestations of liver fire, such as distending pain in the head, irritability and irascibility, flushed face, dream-disturbed sleep and taut pulse. Deficiency types are usually seen in chronic cases, in which the exuberance of liver *yang* is secondary to the deficiency of *yin*.

3. Hypochondriac pain. Pain in the hypochondriac region is usually related to liver disorders. Not only do stagnation of liver *qi* and its complication — blood stasis — cause hypochondriac pain, the accumulation of damp-heat in the liver and gallbladder also has the same effect. Hypochondriac pain caused by stagnation of liver *qi* is distending in property, and is often precipitated or aggravated by the sulks. Pain caused by blood stasis is pricking in character and fixed in location, and may be accompanied by hepatomegaly or splenomegaly. That caused by damp-heat is often associated with bitterness in the mouth, anorexia, nausea, vomiting or jaundice.

4. Mass formation. Either *qi* stagnation or blood stasis due to dysfunction of the liver may cause masses to form. Masses formed by stagnation of *qi* usually have no definite shape.

They come and go unpredictably, accompanied by pain without fixed location. The mass felt in the abdomen due to intestinal spasms is an example of this condition. On the contrary, masses formed by blood stasis, e.g., hepato-splenomegaly or a gynecological tumour, are usually of definited shape and accompanied by localized pain and tenderness.

5. Jaundice. According to traditional Chinese medicine, jaundice occurs when secretion of the bile is impaired. Jaundice is of two types: *yang*-jaundice and *yin*-jaundice. In *yin*-jaundice, cold-damp produced by an impaired spleen and stomach impedes the secretion of bile. In *yang*-jaundice damp-heat caused by an exogenous pathogenic factor or a pathogenic factor produced interiorly by the spleen and stomach after eating bad food or drinking large amounts of alcohol, attacks the liver and gallbladder and impairs bile secretion. *Yang*-jaundice is a disease of short duration marked by bright yellow discoloration of the skin and the sclera. *Yin*-jaundice is a chronic disease characterized by dim yellow discoloration of the skin and the sclera. Since jaundice involves not only the liver and gallbladder but also the spleen and stomach, it is often accompanied by digestive disturbances.

7. Tremors. Tremors, usually involving the distal segments of the limbs, are a symptom of wind. In most cases, deficiency of liver *yin* or deficiency of both liver *yin* and kidney *yin* leads to a nutritional disturbance of the distal muscles causing involuntary shaking or trembling. This is particularly common in the aged. In some cases, deficiency of *qi* and blood which impairs the nutrition of the distal muscles causes tremors. An attack of phlegm-heat after an emotional upset which gives rise to excessive liver fire and which impairs the spleen may also cause tremors. In these cases, the dysfunctioning spleen produces phlegm. Therefore, tremors are closely related to liver troubles, and can be classified into two categories: deficiency type, as occurs in deficiency of liver; excess type, as occurs in excessive liver fire.

8. Convulsions. Convulsions characterized by violent involuntary muscular contractions are also a wind symptom. Excessive heat can lead to convulsions by precipitating liver wind, by consuming body fluids or by penetrating into the "pericardium" (a term used to describe the center of the nervous system). Convulsions can also occur when there is deficiency of *qi* and blood (particularly after massive hemorrhage) and when stagnated blood or turbid phlegm obstruct meridians and collaterals. Therefore, convulsions can occur in many morbid conditions other than liver troubles.

# DIFFERENTIATION OF SYNDROMES

## I. Deficiency syndromes of the liver

Deficiency syndromes of the liver involve shortness of blood and *yin*. When the blood stored in the liver is insufficient, pallor, dizziness, blurring of the vision, dryness of the eyes, and tremors, spasms or numbness of the limbs result, as well as scanty menstrual flow with prolonged cycle in women. If vital essence or fluid of the liver is insufficient, dizziness, blurring of the vision and dryness of the eyes, mouth and throat occur. Tremors, spasms or numbness of the limbs may also appear. Obviously, there are many similarities between the clinical manifestations of these two syndromes. Men who exhibit pallor with pale tongue and women who exhibit decreased menstrual flow should be diagnosed as having deficiency of the liver blood. If patients have no pale complexion, their tongues are somewhat reddened instead of pale and the symptoms of dryness are marked, particularly if there are symptoms showing exuberance of *yang*, the diagnosis should be deficiency of liver *yin*. However, if exuberance of *yang* is marked, the diagnosis should be deficiency of liver *yin* with exuberance of *yang*. When deficiency of liver blood and deficiency of liver *yin* occur simultaneously, the diagnosis is deficiency of liver *yin*-blood.

Deficiency of liver *qi* is seldom diagnosed in isolation. It is usually associated with deficiency of blood. The chief symptoms of deficiency of liver *qi* are lack of strength, tinnitus, impaired hearing and susceptibility to fright.

Insufficiency of liver *yang* may also occur. Its manifestations are depression, cowardliness and cold limbs. This syndrome is rarely seen and hence of little clinical significance.

## II. Excess syndromes of the liver

Excessive emotional changes (especially repressed anger) or exogenous factors (such as damp-heat) cause excess syndromes of the liver. Mental irritation can cause depression syndrome or stagnation of liver *qi* syndrome. They are manifested by irritability or irascibility and distension and pain in the regions where the Liver Merdian traverses, such as hypochondriac, mammary, lateral pectoral and lower abdominal regions. In addition, the patient may complain of a choking sensation. When stagnated *qi* combines with phlegm, the choking sensation becomes more marked, as if there were a lump obstructing the throat. This is known as "plum plug" (globus hystericus). In women, stagnation of liver *qi* often leads to irregular menstruation. If stagnated *qi* influences the spleen and stomach, digestive symptoms, such as anorexia, belching, regurgitation, loose stool and abdominal distension, will result. Uncomplicated depression of liver *qi* is diagnosed only when digestive symptoms are mild. If digestive symptoms are manifest, the diagnosis should be disharmony of the liver with the stomach or spleen or both. Depression of liver *qi* often occurs in neurosis and menstrual disorders.

As stated by Zhu Danxi in *Danxi's Experimental Therapy* (1481), "Excessive *qi* (energy) gives rise to fire." Over-stagnation of *qi* may transform into fire syndrome. The fire of the liver usually flares up along the Liver and Gallbladder Meridians reaching the head, eyes and ears, causing headache, dizziness, bloodshot eyes, tinnitus and impairment of hearing. Since these symptoms also occur in deficiency syndromes, such as deficiency of *yin* of the liver or the kidneys, further differentiation is necessary.

There are two kinds of liver fire or exuberance of liver *yang*. One is of excess type, the other of deficiency type. The fire of excess type is usually acute at onset and is precipitated by an emotional upset, while the fire or exuberance of *yang* of deficiency type occurs, as a rule, secondarily to deficiency of *yin*, and is hence characterized by various manifestations of *yin* deficiency in addition to symptoms of fire or exuberance of liver *yang*.

An extreme liver fire of excess type may produce wind syndromes manifested by convulsions and sudden loss of consciousness accompanied by hemiplegia. However, deficiency of blood may also cause wind syndromes, but these are characterized by tremors. In the former wind syndromes, the onset is acute or sudden, while in the latter the course of the disease is always chronic.

# COMMON SYNDROMES IN INTERNAL MEDICINE

## I. Deficiency syndromes of the liver

**1. Deficiency of blood in the liver** (occurring in hepatitis, neurosis, anemia, menstrual disorders)

Primary manifestations: Dizziness, blurring of vision, dryness of eyes, tremors, spasms, numbness of limbs, scanty menstrual flow with prolonged cycle, pallor, pale tongue and thready pulse.

Principle of treatment: Enrich the blood in the liver.

Formula of choice: Si Wu Tang (Decoction of Four Ingredients).

**2. Deficiency of *yin* of the liver with exuberance of *yang*** (occurring in hepatitis, neurosis, hypertension)

Primary manifestations: Symptoms of blood deficiency of the liver (except pallor and pale tongue) plus dry mouth and throat, scanty tongue coating and taut, thready pluse; feverishness of the palms and soles, accompanied by marked dizziness, headache, tinnitus, reddened tongue with little coating and taut, thready and rapid pulse indicates deficiency of liver *yin* with exuberance of *yang*.

Principle of treatment: Nourish liver *yin*; if there is exuberance of *yang*, nourish liver *yin* and suppress hyperactive *yang*.

Formula of choice: For deficiency of liver *yin*, Yiguan Jian (Ever-effective Decoction for Nourishing the Liver and Kidneys); for deficiency of liver *yin* with exuberance of *yang*, Qi Ju Dihuang Wan (Bolus of Rehmannia with Wolfberry and Chrysanthemum).

**3. Stagnation of liver *qi*** (occurring in neurosis, hepatitis, cholecystitis, irregular menstruation)

Primary manifestations: Irritability and irascibility, distension and pain in the hypochondriac, mammary, lateral pectoral or lower abdominal regions where the Liver Meridian traverses, discomfort in the chest, frequent sighing, irregular menstruation in women and taut pulse.

Principle of treatment: Relieve the stagnation of liver *qi*.

Formula of choice: Chaihu Shugan San (Bupleurum Powder for Soothing the Liver).

**4. Flaming-up of liver fire** (occurring in hypertension, Meniere's syndrome, acute conjunctivitis, hemorrhage of the upper digestive tract)

Primary manifestations: Marked irascibility, headache and dizziness, bloodshot eyes, tinnitus, impairment of hearing, taut rapid pulse and reddened tongue with yellow coating; sudden onset of hemorrhage, such as hematemesis or epistaxis, may also occur.

Principle of treatment: Purge the liver of fire.

Formula of choice: Longdan Xiegan Tang (Decoction of Gentian for Purging Liver Fire).

**5. Stirring-up of the liver wind**

Primary manifestations:

(1) Transformation of exuberant liver fire into wind (occurring in cerebrovascular accidents): Sudden onset of syncope, convulsions or apoplexy accompanied by hemiplegia, reddened tongue and taut, rapid pulse.

Principle of treatment: Subdue the liver fire and calm the wind.

Formula of choice: Zhen'gan Xifeng Tang (Decoction for Tranquilizing Liver-Wind).

(2) Production of internal wind due to extreme heat (occurring in encephalitis, meningitis and other infectious diseases with high fever): Convulsions and opisthotonos during high fever.

Principle of treatment: Clear away intense heat and toxic substances.

Formula of choice: Qingwen Baidu Yin (Antipyretic and Antitoxic Decoction).

(3) Production of internal wind due to deficiency of blood (occurring in some chronic neurological diseases): Tremors or numbness of limbs, involuntary head shaking, pale tongue and taut, thready pulse.

Principle of treatment: Nourish the blood and calm the wind.

Formula of choice: Bugan Tang (Decoction for Replenishing the Liver).

**6. Damp-heat in the liver and gallbladder** (occurring in icteric jaundice, acute cholecystitis, cholelithiasis)

Primary manifestations: Pain or colic in the right hypochondriac region, jaundice, bitter taste in the mouth, nausea, vomiting, abdominal distension, yellow sticky or greasy coating of the tongue and taut and rapid pulse.

Principle of treatment: Clear the liver and gallbladder of damp-heat.

Formula of choice: Yinchenhao Tang (Oriental Wormwood Decoction).

## Section 2   SYNDROMES OF THE HEART AND THE SMALL INTESTINE

The heart controls blood and vessels, and houses the mind. The small intestine assimilates the essence from food and rejects the dross. Since the spleen controls the whole process of digestion, syndromes of the small intestine with digestive symptoms are often considered syndromes of the spleen. The heart and the small intestine are discussed together because meridians connect them, thus they are related.

## SYMPTOMS AND SIGNS

### I. Symptoms due to dysfunction of the heart in housing the mind

One is full of vigor and has normal consciousness when the function of the heart in housing the mind is normal. If this function is in disorder, neurotic symptoms or impairment of consciousness may occur. Various etiological and pathogenetic factors may disrupt this function. For instance, vital essence and blood in the heart provide the material basis for housing the mind; if either one is deficient, the mind will have in effect, no place to reside in. It will wander. The patient will be absentminded or distracted, and will experience memory lapses, palpitations and fidgetiness in the daytime and insomnia and dream-disturbed sleep at night.

Pathogenic factors, such as fire and phlegm, may also impair the heart's function. Fire prevents the mind from residing in peace and causes it to wander. Manifestations in these cases are similar to those seen in cases in which a deficiency of vital essence and blood disturb the heart's ability to house the mind. However, these syndromes are different in nature: syndromes due to interference by fire are often of excess type, while those due to deficiency of vital essence and blood are always of deficiency type.

Phlegm may mist the heart, impairing consciousness and causing drowsiness, blurring of the mind or even coma. If phlegm-fire attacks the heart, the manifestations will be both the impairment of consciousness and the wandering of the mind, as seen in mental restlessness with incoherent speech or mania.

The functional disorders of the heart in housing the mind and the consequent symptoms are summarized in Table VI-I.

**Table VI-I. Functional Disorders of the Heart in Housing the Mind**

|  | Pathology | Symptoms |
|---|---|---|
| Failure in housing the mind | Deficiency of *qi* | Wandering of the mind |
|  | Deficiency of blood | (absentmindedness, insomnia, |
|  | Interference by fire | dream-disturbed sleep, etc.) |
| Misting of the heart | Interference by phlegm-fire | Derangement of the mind (mental restlessness, mania, etc.) |
|  | Interference by phlegm or damp-phlegm | Blurring of the mind (drowsiness or even coma) |

## II. Symptoms due to dysfunction of the heart in controlling blood and vessels

Heart *qi* (energy) gives the blood the motive force it requires to circulate through the vessels. If heart *qi* is insufficient, cardiac palpitations, shortness of breath and thready and feeble pulse result. Sometimes, deficiency of heart *qi* may impair the regular rhythm of the heartbeat, causing arrhythmia. Deficiency of heart *qi* may further result in blood stasis. Stagnation of blood in the vessels of the heart itself usually causes precordial or substernal pain, transient in mild cases and persistent in severe cases accompanied by cyanosis, purplish tongue or tongue with purple spots. In addition, either deficiency of heart *qi* or deficiency of blood impairs the blood supply throughout the body, the most conspicuous manifestation of which is pallor, including pale complexion and pale tongue.

Symptoms due to disorders of the heart in controlling blood and vessels are summarized in Table VI-II.

**Table VI-II. Functional Disorders of the Heart in Controlling Blood and Vessels**

|  | Pathology | Symtoms |
|---|---|---|
| Deficiency of heart *qi* (energy) | Insufficient activity of the heart | Palpitations, shortness of breath, pallor, pale tongue |
|  | Irregular issue of the impulse for the heartbeat | Arrythmia |
|  | Stagnated flow of *qi* and blood in the heart vessel | Precordial pain, cyanosis, purplish tongue |
| Deficiency of blood in the heart | Insufficient blood supply for circulation | Pallor, pale tongue, dizziness |

Other manifestations may also appear when the heart is diseased. The tongue is taken as the window of the heart. Although various diseases may change the tongue, diseases of the heart are frequently reflected in the tongue. A pale tongue means a deficiency of *qi* and/or blood of the heart; a purplish tongue is a sign of blood stasis; a reddened tongue, particularly a reddened tongue tip with ulcerations, is characteristic of hyperactivity (flaring-up) of heart fire. Fire of the heart can either flare up or shift downwards. In the latter case, the fire causes urethral pain, burning sensation during micturition and even hematuria.

Following is a discussion of several common symptoms of a diseased heart:

1. Palpitations. Palpitations may be due to disturbance of the heart (mind) by emotional factors (such as fright), insufficiency of heart *qi* or blood, deficiency of heart *yin* with exuberance of heart fire or exhaustion of heart *yang*. A patient with palpitations due to disturbance of the mind is apt to be frightened and suffer from insomnia. Palpitations due to insufficiency of heart *qi*, usually occurring during physical exertion and subsiding after resting, are often accompanied by shortness of breath, dizziness, weakness and spontaneous sweating. Irritability, fidgetiness, dizziness and insomnia accompany palpitations caused by deficiency of heart *yin* with exuberance of fire. Palpitations that occur when heart *yang* is exhausted are associated with dyspnea, cold limbs, edema and oliguria.

2. Insomnia. Normally, the heart (mind) controls sleep. When *yang-qi* (physical and mental activity) turns from movement to rest, one falls asleep, and when it turns from rest to movement, one awakes. Therefore, normal sleep is based on the natural rhythmic change of *yin* and *yang*. Insomnia is a common symptom of a break in this rhythm.

Although dysfunction of the heart in housing the mind is the main cause of insomnia, derangement of other *zang-fu* organs may also impair the rhythmic change of *yin-yang*. Thus, insomnia is a common symptom in the following syndromes:

(1) Deficiency syndrome of both the heart and the spleen characterized by dream-disturbed sleep, palpitations, forgetfulness, lassitude, anorexia and pallor.

(2) Deficiency of *yin* with exuberance of heart fire or liver fire or both, marked by fidgetiness, insomnia, dizziness, tinnitus, dryness in the mouth, hot sensation in the palms and soles and reddened tongue with rapid pulse; there may also be nocturnal emissions, forgetfulness, palpitations and aching in the loins.

(3) Disturbance of heart by phlegm-fire marked by insomnia, a feeling of stuffiness in the chest, heaviness of the head, fidgetiness, bitter taste in the mouth, dizziness, yellow and greasy tongue coating and slippery, rapid pulse.

## DIFFERENTIATION OF SYNDROMES

I. Deficiency syndromes of the heart are classified into four categories, deficiency of *qi*, *yang*, blood and *yin*. *Qi* pertains to *yang* and blood to *yin*, so deficiency syndromes of the heart can be more generally grouped into two categories: deficiency of blood and *yin*, and deficiency of *qi* and *yang*. The former is characterized by nervous symptoms (usually seen in neurosis or general debility). This is because a lack of material basis causes a functional disorder of the heart in housing the mind. The latter is manifested by cardiovascular insufficiency, as a result of a diminishing of the dynamic force responsible for blood circulation.

Either deficiency of heart blood or deficiency of heart *yin* causes "wandering of the mind" manifested by fidgetiness, insomnia and dream-disturbed sleep. Symptoms help differentiate between these two syndromes. Deficiency of heart blood is marked by pallor, pale tongue and other manifestations indicating insufficient blood supply. Deficiency of heart *yin*, on the other hand, is accompanied by symptoms of endogenous heat. If endogenous heat symptoms include lowgrade fever, malar flush, feverish sensation in the chest, palms and soles, night sweating and reddened tongue with little coating, the condition is deficiency of heart *yin* with exuberance of endogenous heat or fire.

Both deficiency syndromes of heart *qi* and of heart *yang* share diminished functional activity of the heart as their common feature. The only difference is that deficiency of *qi* displays no cold manifestations, while deficiency of *yang* is accompanied by cold symptoms, such as chilliness, aversion to cold and cold limbs. In other words, deficiency of heart *yang* equals deficiency of heart *qi* plus endogenous cold. If deficiency of heart *yang* occurs suddenly or reaches an extreme, collapse or even shock may occur.

## II. Excess syndromes of the heart

Fire, phlegm and stagnated blood, which in most cases are endogenous due to internal injury, commonly invade the heart. Exogenous pathogenic heat may cause high fever with impairment of consciousness or even coma, but it is customarily called invasion of the pericardium by evil heat rather than invasion of the heart.

Hyperactivity (fire) of the heart can cause three groups of symptoms: (1) those caused by flaming of the fire in the heart, such as fidgetiness with feverish sensation, insomnia and restlessness; (2) those due to a flare-up of the fire with pain and ulceration of the tongue as the chief manifestations; and (3) those in which the fire shifts downward, marked by urodynia and hematuria. All three groups of symptoms may appear individually or simultaneously.

Invasion of the heart by phlegm or phlem-fire causes abnormal responsiveness of the mind. Phlegm alone usually results in inhibitory symptoms, such as impaired consciousness or even coma, as seen in apoplexy. Phlegm combined with fire often causes abnormal excitation, as seen in hysteria, schizophrenia or manic psychosis.

Blood stasis in the heart vessels implies that local accumulation of stagnated blood is the pathogenic factor. The syndrome it causes is naturally of excess type. However, in most cases deficiency of *qi* or *yang* of the heart causes blood stasis, so it is actually a complicated syndrome of deficiency and excess. The mild syndrome is often seen in angina pectoris, the severe one in myocardial infarction.

## COMMON SYNDROMES IN INTERNAL MEDICINE

**1. Deficiency of blood of the heart** (occurring in neurosis, anemia and some debilitated states)

Primary manifestations: Palpitations and fidgetiness, insomnia, dream-disturbed sleep, hypomnesia, pallor, pale tongue and deep and thready pulse.

Principle of treatment: Tonify the blood of the heart.

Formula of choice: Siwu Tang (Decoction of Four Ingredients).

**2. Deficiency of heart *yin*** (occurring in neurosis and various consumptive diseases).

Primary manifestations: Palpitations and fidgetiness, insomnia, dream-disturbed sleep, hypomnesia, reddened tongue and thready, rapid pulse; in some cases, low-grade fever, malar flush, feverish sensation in palms and soles and night sweating due to exuberant fire secondary to *yin* deficiency.

Principle of treatment: Replenish *yin* of the heart and induce tranquilization.

Formula of choice: Tianwang Buxin Dan (Cardiotonic pill).

**3. Deficiency of heart *qi*** (occurring in various heart diseases with cardiac insufficiency)

Primary manifestations: Palpitations and shortness of breath aggravated upon exertion, feeling of oppression in the chest, spontaneous sweating, pallor, pale tongue, and thready and feeble pulse or arrhythmia.

Principle of treatment: Reinforce heart *qi*.

Formula of choice: Si Junzi Tang (Decoction of Four Noble Drugs).

**4. Deficiency of heart *yang*** (occurring in various heart diseases with cardiac insufficiency)

Primary manifestations: Symptoms of deficiency of heart *qi*, together with aversion to cold and cold limbs.

Principle of treatment: Warm and tonify the heart.

Formula of choice: Si Junzi Tang (Decoction of Four Noble Drugs) plus aconite and cinnamon twigs.

**5. Collapes of heart-*yang*** (occurring in shock)

Primary manifestations: Profuse cold sweating, fainting or loss of consciousness, extremely cold limbs and scarcely perceptible pulse.

Principle of treatment: Restore *yang* and relieve collapse.

Formula of choice: Shen Fu Tang (Decoction of Ginseng and Prepared Aconite).

**6. Hyperactivity of heart fire** (occurring in stress with glossitis, ulcer of tongue or some urological diseases)

Primary manifestations: Insomnia and fidgetiness, thirst and bitter taste in the mouth, ulceration and pain of the tongue with reddened tip and yellow coating and rapid pulse; in some cases, burning pain in the urethra during micturition and passage of hot and dark urine or even hematuria.

Principle of treatment: Clear the heart of excessive fire.

Formula of choice: Daochi San (Powder for Treating Dark Urine).

**7. Stagnation of blood in the heart vessels** (occurring in angina pectoris and myocardial infarction)

Primary manifestations: Precordial or substernal pain (transient pricking or severe colicky, referring to the shoulder and arm), dark purplish tongue or purple spots on the tongue and deep, hesitant pulse or arrhythmia.

Principle of treatment: Remove stagnation from the heart vessels.

Formula of choice: Gualou Xiebai Baijiu Tang (Decoction of Trichosanthes and Allium with Wine).

## Section 3    SYNDROMES OF THE SPLEEN AND THE STOMACH

The spleen and the stomach form the system of digestion and absorption and provide the material basis of the acquired constitution.

The spleen digests food, transports, distributes and transforms nutrients and replenishes *qi*. The latter function promotes water metabolism and keeps the blood flowing within the blood vessels. The spleen sends nutrients upward to the heart and lungs and keeps *qi* moving upward.

The stomach receives food, transforms it into chyme and sends the preliminarily digested food downward into the intestines.

Since the spleen and the stomach are so closely related, they are often considered together, particularly in digestive disorders. It should be noted, however, that the spleen performs more functions than just digestion.

## SYMPTOMS AND SIGNS

Impairment of the spleen function in digesting food usually results in indigestion which is marked by anorexia, abdominal distension and diarrhea. Impairment of the spleen function in transportation, distribution and transformation of nutrients leads to lassitude, emaciation and sallow complexion. Replenishing *qi* is closely related with the transportation, distribution and transformation of nutrients. Therefore, an impaired spleen is one of the main causes of general deficiency of *qi*, which is manifested as listlessness, lack of strength, shortness of breath and feeble pulse.

Impairment of the spleen function in distributing fluids and promoting water metabolism leads to retention of water (damp) in the body. This causes various symptoms depending on the location of the damp retained. A stuffy sensation in the chest with nausea and vomiting results when the damp is retained in the chest and epigastric region; diarrhea occurs when the damp is retained in the intestines; pleural effusion or ascites occurs if the damp is retained in the corresponding body cavity; edema appears when the damp is retained subcutaneously; and asthenia with heavy sensation of the limbs results if damp is retained in the extremities. Therefore, the *Canon of Medicine* says that "various endogenous dampness and water retention are related to the spleen." Damp retained in the lungs may become condensed and turn into phlegm which, in turn, causes cough and asthma. Thus, in chronic cases, the spleen is the source of phlegm.

If the spleen fails to keep the blood flowing within the blood vessels, various kinds of chronic hemorrhage may occur, such as uterine bleeding, hematochezia and hematuria. In a chronic case of spleen insufficiency when the spleen fails to keep the nutrients and *qi* going upwards, prolonged diarrhea, prolapse of the rectum and uterus, gastroptosis and other visceroptosis will occur, all of which are called "sinking" symptoms.

Reduction of the stomach function in receiving food causes loss of appetite and reduces food intake. Indigestion is the most common disorder caused by diminished stomach function. On the contrary, hyperactivity of the stomach in exuberance of stomach fire often leads to polyphagia.

A normally functioning stomach sends its contents downwards. An upward perversion causes nausea, vomiting, belching and hiccups. Gastralgia is also a common symptom in stomach diseases.

Following is a detailed discussion of common symptoms of stomach diseases.

(1) Nausea and vomiting. An upward perversion of the stomach function causes vomiting. Nausea has a similar pathogenesis, but it is less severe. They often occur together, the former a prodrome of the latter.

Vomiting can be divided into two main types: excess and deficiency. Vomiting of excess type has an acute onset and short course, resulting from exogenous affections of the stomach, stagnation of undigested food in the stomach due to improper diet, accumulation of phlegm and fluid in the stomach or attack of the stomach by liver *qi* after an emotional upset. Vomiting of deficiency type due to reduced functioning of the spleen and stomach in digesting and transporting their contents has a gradual onset and prolonged course. The vomitus provides significant clues for diagnosis. Vomiting sour and foul contents indicates stagnation of undigested food in the stomach; vomiting mucus and liquid suggests accumulation of phlegm and fluid in the stomach; repeated retching with little or no vomitus is a sign of deficiency of stomach *yin*.

(2) Hiccups. Hiccups result from upward perversion in the stomach's function. In most cases, they are transient, need no medication and have little clinical significance. But in some cases, they persist and indicate a problem when they occur during the course of a serious disease.

Persistent hiccups can be categorized based on the general parameters of excess versus deficiency and cold versus heat. Hiccups of excess-cold type are low-pitched and forcible and can be alleviated by warmth, indicating cold in the stomach. Hiccups of excess-heat type are loud, forcible and continuous and are accompanied by foul breath and constipation, indicating the presence of stomach fire. Hiccups of deficiency-cold type are weak and low-pitched with interruptions and are often accompanied by cold limbs and general weakness, indicating deficiency of spleen *yang*. Hiccups of deficiency-heat type are hasty with interruptions and are usually accompanied by thirst and dryness of the mouth and throat, indicating deficiency of stomach *yin*.

(3) Acid regurgitation. The stomach affected by stagnated liver fire and the spleen and stomach affected by deficiency-cold are the main causes of acid regurgitation. Thus, acid regurgitation is of two types: heat and cold. The former is accompanied by fidgetiness, bitterness in the mouth and taut rapid pulse, the latter by distension in the epigastrium, belching and white tongue coating.

(4) Gastralgia. Atmospheric changes (particularly cold), irregular meals, improper diet, emotional upsets and overfatigue are among the causes of gastralgia. Gastralgia has the same pathogenic basis as any other pain, i.e., obstruction of the flow of *qi* and blood. Gastralgia can be divided into several categories: (a) gastralgia due to pathogenic cold, characterized by sudden onset of severe pain in the stomach that can be alleviated by warmth; (b) gastralgia due to stagnated food, accompanied by foul belching, acid regurgitation and thick greasy tongue coating that is alleviated after vomiting; (c) gastralgia due to an attack of the stomach by liver *qi* during a fit of the sulks, the pain

being distending in character, referring to the hypochondriac regions and accompanied by frequent belching; (d) gastralgia occurring in deficiency-cold syndrome of the spleen and stomach that is mild but lingering and can be relieved by pressure and warmth; and (e) gastralgia caused by blood stasis, characterized by stabbing or pricking pain fixed in location and sometimes accompanied by hematemesis or tarry stools.

(5) Belching. Belching occurs in the following syndromes: (a) stagnation of undigested food in the stomach, occurring frequently after eating and accompanied by sour and foul gas and sometimes associated with nausea, vomiting and thick turbid tongue coating; (b) accumulation of phlegm-fire in the stomach due to improper diet, in which belching is accompanied by stuffiness in the chest and sometimes by vomiting of phlegm and yellow, greasy coating of the tongue; (c) disharmony of the liver and the stomach, in which belching is often accompanied by abdominal distension and precipitated or aggravated by fits of the sulks; and (d) deficiency-cold of the spleen and the stomach, in which belching occurs on and off and is accompanied by general weakness, cold limbs, lusterless complexion and regurgitation of fluid.

(6) Diarrhea. Diarrhea in disorders of the spleen and stomach involves frequent loose stools which may contain undigested food but no pus or blood. If there is passage of pus or blood with the stools, the diarrhea is usually due to invasion of the large intestine by damp-heat (acute dysentery).

Diarrhea may be encountered in the following conditions: In acute cases, it is caused by exogenous pathogenic factors (particularly cold-damp and damp-heat that impair the function of the spleen and stomach) or imporper diet; in chronic cases, diarrhea is due to diminished function of the spleen and stomach, deficiency of kidney *yang*, or attack of the spleen by liver *qi*. Diarrhea caused by cold-damp is characterized by loose or even watery stools and white, greasy tongue coating and is often accompanied by colds (stuffy nose, headache, chilliness and mild fever). Diarrhea caused by damp-heat is due to improper diet and is marked by foul watery stool with abdominal pain, heat sensation in the anus, thirst and yellow, greasy tongue coating. Diarrhea due to overfeeding is characterized by stools that smell like putrid eggs and is accompanied by abdominal distention and pain which is alleviated after bowel movement and by belching of sour and foul gas. A dirty greasy tongue coating is also characteristic.

Chronic diarrhea due to diminished function of the spleen and stomach is characterized by recurrence of diarrhea with stools containing undigested food, usually aggravated by a heavy meal, and accompanied by anorexia, epigastric distension after meal, sallow complexion and pale tongue with whitish coating. In chronic diarrhea due to deficiency of kidney *yang*, persistent diarrhea occurs before dawn and is accompanied by borborygmi and periumbilical colic which is alleviated after defecation, as well as cold limbs and aversion to cold, especially cold to the abdomen. If chronic diarrhea is due to an attack of the spleen by liver *qi*, repeated diarrhea occurs after emotional stimuli that impair the normal flow of liver *qi*, and this condition is accompanied by a stuffy sensation in the chest and hypochondriac regions, belching, loss of appetite and abdominal pain immediately before defecation.

# DIFFERENTIATION OF SYNDROMES

## I. Deficiency syndromes of the spleen

Deficiency syndromes of the spleen refer to an insufficiency in its function rather than a decrease in its material constituents. The fundamental condition of various deficiency syndromes of the spleen is deficiency of spleen *qi*, which diminishes the spleen's ability to digest and assimilate. If this condition persists over a considerable length of time, the patient's strength and vitality will be impaired. Deficiency of spleen *qi* (hypofunction of the spleen) may cause any of a series of deficiency syndromes to develop. If deficiency of spleen *qi* is accompanied by "cold manifestations," such as aversion to cold and abdominal pain aggravated by cold, the diagnosis is deficiency of spleen *yang*. If deficiency of spleen *qi* is accompanied by symptoms indicating retention of dampness manifested as diarrhea, leukorrhagia with profuse thin discharge, edema of the limbs and thick slippery tongue coating, the diagnosis is hypofunction of the spleen with retention of dampness. If deficiency of *qi* is marked by the spleen failing to keep the nutrients and *qi* moving upward, sinking of spleen *qi* will occur, marked by prolonged lienteric diarrhea or various kinds of visceroptosis.

The spleen's role in keeping the blood circulating within the vessels is also associated with spleen *qi*. So, deficiency of spleen *qi* may lead to bleeding. Bleeding due to deficiency of spleen *qi* is characterized by chronicity and occurrence in the lower part of the body, as seen in excessive menstrual flow, recurrent hematochezia and persistent hematuria.

The formation of general *qi* and blood is closely related to the spleen, which supplies the essential elements for *qi* generation and hemopoiesis. Therefore, in severe hypofunction of the spleen, not only does deficiency of general *qi* marked by lassitude and fatigability occur but also deficiency of blood. However, unlike the liver which stores blood and the heart which contains blood, the spleen is not a special blood container; deficiency of blood in the spleen, if it occurs, is merely a part of general blood deficiency and therefore requires no special stress in the diagnosis.

Deficiency of spleen *yin* refers to a shortness of fluids, usually manifested as constipation.

## II. Excess syndromes of the spleen

Among the pathogenic factors that attack the spleen, damp is the most common. It may originate from outside as an atmospheric factor or be produced within the body as a result of irregular food intake. Cold-damp often invades the spleen after one is chilled by rain or overeats raw and cold food. Because exogenous cold-damp impairs the transporting and transforming functions, it may cause a syndrome very similar to hypofunction of the spleen with stagnation of damp. Cold-damp syndromes are of excess origin, usually occurring after an apparent etiological event and having an acute onset, while hypofunction of the spleen with stagnation of damp is of deficiency origin, often found in chronic cases, in which the symptoms of hypofunction of the spleen precede the damp manifestations.

When damp-heat invades the spleen, it has a clinical picture similar to that of damp-heat invading the liver and gallbladder. Both syndromes may be seen in acute icteric hepatitis and cholecystitis. However, damp-heat in the liver and gall bladder displays hypochondriac pain and jaundice but few digestive disorders, while damp-heat in the spleen is marked by prominent digestive disorders but no hypochondriac pain.

### III. Deficiency syndromes of the stomach

The deficiency syndromes of the stomach include deficiency of *qi*, *yang* and *yin* of the stomach. Deficiency of stomach *qi* (diminished function of the stomach) is manifested by loss of appetite and reduced food intake. It is difficult to differentiate deficiency of stomach *qi* from deficiency of spleen *qi*, since both of them involve impairment of digestion. Deficiency of stomach *qi* usually entails epigastric pain, eructation, belching, nausea and vomiting, while deficiency of spleen typically manifests itself as abdominal pain, loose stools, lassitude, emaciation and general weakness.

Deficiency of stomach *yang* can be stated as deficiency of stomach *qi* plus cold manifestations. Thus, gastralgia due to deficiency of stomach *qi* can be alleviated by pressure or food, while gastralgia due to deficiency of *yang* is alleviated by warmth.

Deficiency of stomach *yin* is a common syndrome characterized by insufficient fluids in the digestive tract. However, the difficulty in determining whether the constipation due to deficiency of fluids is of spleen or stomach origin ("stomach" in traditional Chinese medicine sometimes refers to the whole digestive tract) has led some authors to avoid any mention of "deficiency of spleen *yin*."

## COMMON SYNDROMES IN INTERNAL MEDICINE

**1. Deficiency of spleen and stomach *qi*** (occurring in peptic ulcer, chronic gastritis, chronic colitis, functional disorders of the gastrointestinal system, chronic hepatitis and other digestive diseases)

Primary manifestations:

(1) Weakness of the stomach: Poor appetite, reduced food intake, epigastric pain alleviated by food or pressure, belching and acid eructation or nausea and vomiting.

(2) Weakness of the spleen: Anorexia, fullness and stuffy feeling in the epigastrium after eating, abdominal distension, loose bowels or edema, pale, plump and tender tongue with whitish coating and teeth prints at its borders and soft and weak pulse; in chronic case, sallow complexion, general weakness, lassitude and emaciation.

Principle of treatment: Strengthen the spleen and regulate the stomach.

Formula of choice: Xiangsha Liujunzi Tang (Decoction of Auklandia and Amomum with Six Noble Ingredients) for syndrome in which weakness of the stomach predominates; Shen Ling Baizhu San (Powder of Ginseng, Poria and White Atractylodes) for syndrome in which weakness of the spleen predominates.

**2. Deficiency of spleen and stomach *yang*, deficiency-cold syndrome of the spleen and the stomach** (occurring in peptic ulcer, chronic gastritis, chronic colitis, functional derangements of the gastrointestinal tract, chronic hepatitis, liver cirrhosis)

Primary manifestations: Symptoms of deficiency of spleen and stomach *qi* aggravated by cold and accompanied by other cold manifestations (aversion to cold, cold limbs), pale tongue with white slippery coating and deep, feeble pulse; other possible symptoms in deficiency of spleen *yang* cases include chronic diarrhea, edema with oliguria and excessive leukorrhea with thin discharge.

Principle of treatment: Warm and tonify the spleen and stomach.

Formula of choice: Xiao Jianzhong Tang (Minor Decoction for Strengthening the Middle-*jiao*).

**3. Sinking of spleen *qi*, sinking of middle-*jiao* qi** (occurring in chronic colitis, functional disorders of the intestines, prolapse of rectum or uterus, gastroptosis and other visceroptosis)

Primary manifestations: Deficiency of *qi* (or *yang*) of the spleen plus chronic diarrhea, drippling of urine after urination, prolapse of rectum or uterus and symptoms of other viscerptosis.

Principle of treatment: Lift spleen *qi*.

Formula of choice: Buzhong Yiqi Tang (Decoction for Reinforcing Middle-*jiao* and Replenishing *Qi*)

**4. Failure of the spleen to control blood** (occurring in various kinds of chronic bleeding, e.g., functional uterine bleeding and hematochezia, and hemorrhagic diseases, e.g., thrombocytopenic purpura, allergic purpura)

Primary manifestations: Menorrhagia, hematochezia, hematuria, subcutaneous hemorrhage and other bleeding (usually chronic), pale tongue and thready weak pulse.

Principle of treatment: Reinforce spleen *qi* and arrest bleeding.

Formula of choice: Guipi Tang (Decoction for Restoration of the Spleen).

**5. Deficiency of stomach *yin*** (occurring in chronic gastritis, peptic ulcer, dyspepsia)

Primary manifestations: Dryness of the lips and mouth, feeling hungry but with no desire for food, retching, hiccups, epigastric pain and distress, constipation, dry and reddened tongue with scanty coating, and thready rapid pulse.

Principle of treatment: Nourish stomach *yin*.

Formula of choice: Yiwei Tang (Stomach-nourishing Decoction).

**6. Hypofunction of the spleen with stagnation of damp** (occurring in chronic gastritis, chronic colitis, chronic hepatitis, edema, leukorrhagia)

Primary manifestations: Heavy sensation of the head as if it were wrapped, loss of appetite, fullness and distension in the stomach, nausea, diarrhea, edema of the limbs, excessive leukorrhea with thin, whitish discharge, slippery and whitish tongue coating and relaxed pulse.

Principle of treatment: Remove damp and invigorate the spleen.

Formula of choice: Pingwei San (Peptic Powder) in combination with Wuling San (Five Drugs Powder).

**7. Invasion of the spleen by cold-damp** (occurring in acute gastritis, colitis, colds with digestive disorders)

Primary manifestations: Epigastric distension, loss of appetite, sticky sensation in the mouth with no thirst, aversion to cold, edema of limbs, loose stools, whitish, greasy coating of the tongue and relaxed pulse.

Principle of treatment: See Hypofunction of the spleen with stagnation of damp.

Formula of choice: See Hypofunction of the spleen with stagnation of damp.

**8. Invasion of the spleen by damp-heat** (occurring in acute icteric hepatitis, acute cholecystitis)

Primary manifestations: Loss of appetite (particularly no desire for greasy food), nausea and vomiting, epigastric distension, sticky sensation in the mouth or bright yellow discoloration of skin and sclera or leukorrhea with yellow sticky discharge, yellow and greasy tongue coating and soft and rapid pulse.

Principle of treatment: Remove damp-heat.

Formula of choice: Yinchen Wuling San (Powder of Oriental Wormwood and Five Drugs).

**9. Excess of stomach fire** (occurring in febrile stage of certain infectious diseases, diabetes mellitus, aphthosis, gingivitis)

Primary manifestations: Dire thirst, desire for cold drink, polyphagia, foul breath, ulceration in the mouth, swollen and painful gums, constipation or fits of gastralgia with burning sensation, dry and reddened tongue with yellow and thick coating and gigantic or slippery and rapid pulse.

Principle of treatment: Clear the stomach of fire.

Formula of choice: Qingwei San (Powder for Clearing the Stomach of Fire).

**10. Stagnation of undigested food in the stomach** (occurring in dyspepsia)

Primary manifestations: Distension and fullness in the stomach or abdomen, vomiting of fetid substances, belching, acid regurgitation, loss of appetite, constipation or loose bowels with horrid smelling stool, thick greasy coating of the tongue and slippery pulse.

Principle of treatment: Promote digestion and remove the retained food.

Formula of choice: Baohe Wan (Lenitive Pill).

## Section 4    SYNDROMES OF THE LUNGS AND THE LARGE INTESTINE

The lungs control respiration, dominate *qi* and regulate fluid circulation. These functions have a common feature — disseminating and descending, i.e., disseminating *qi* (vital energy) throughout the body and keeping the inspired air and fluids flowing downward. The lungs take the lead in producing acquired *qi*, thus they are closely associated with the body's superficial resistance. In addition, the lungs are the only *zang*-organ that communicates with the exterior, which makes them particularly vulnerable to attacking exogenous pathogenic factors.

The large intestine excretes waste as feces. It is related to the lungs. Thus, many lung diseases of excess type can be satisfactorily treated with cathartics that act on the large intestine.

## SYMPTOMS AND SIGNS

### 1. Symptoms due to impeded respiration

Cough and asthma are the most common symptoms when the disseminating and descending functions of the lungs are disturbed. Exogenous pathogenic factors, such as wind, cold or heat, or endogenous pathogenic factors, such as damp-phlegm from a hypofunctioning spleen or fire from a depressed liver, can impede the air passage, causing these symptoms to emerge.

Expectoration is another common symptom of diseased lungs. Because various pathological factors and changes produce phlegm of different properties, gross examination of the sputum provides important information for differential diagnosis. Thin, whitish sputum suggests the existence of cold; thick or yellow sputum indicates the presence of heat; cough with scanty, thick sputum difficult to expectorate implies dryness; and profuse expectoration suggests dampness. In fact, expectoration is often considered the cause of impeded respiration rather than a resultant symptom.

### 2. Symptoms due to insufficiency in dominating *qi*

Three groups of symptoms indicate lungs that are insufficient in dominating *qi*: (1) shortness of breath, feeble voice and weakness in coughing due to diminished supply of *qi* for the lungs; (2) general weakness and lassitude due to deficiency of *qi* throughout the body; (3) spontaneous sweating and susceptibility to exogenous affection due to weakened superficial defensive power. The first group of symptoms relates specifically to diagnoses of syndromes of the lungs, while the latter two groups have less significance in differential diagnosis since they may also be present when the functional activities of other viscera are insufficient. For example, general weakness and lassitude may occur when the function of the spleen in reinforcing *qi* is impaired; spontaneous sweating occurs when the functional activity of the heart is weakened.

### 3. Symptoms due to disturbance in regulating the water passages

Exogenous pathogenic factors invading the lungs may cause edema. For example, edema appears in acute nephritis after an upper respiratory infection. Traditional Chinese medicine holds that in such a case the pathogenesis of edema is impairment of the function of the lungs in regulating the water passages, which prevents fluids from flowing downwards to the kidneys and on to the urinary bladder. This causes accumulation of fluid in the upper part of the body. Oliguria results, and the edema is more marked in the face and eyelids. Treatment of the lungs with diaphoretics may result in diuresis and subsidence of edema, a therapeutic effect which supports this hypothesis.

Additional discussion of several common symptoms follows.

Cough. Coughs are of two kinds: those caused by exogenous affections and those due to internal injuries. In exogenous affections, cough has an acute onset. In most cases, it occurs as a symptom of catching cold (affection by wind-cold), but various atmospheric factors can result in cough. The common factors are wind, cold, heat and dryness. Cough due to wind-cold is often accompanied by stuffy nose with watery discharge, sneezing, sore throat, expectoration of thin, whitish sputum, headache and chilliness or fever. Wind-heat is marked by cough accompanied by thick, yellowish nasal discharge, sore throat, expectoration of thick, yellowish sputum, headache and fever. Heat in the lungs is characterized by cough accompanied by expectoration of thick or yellow or purulent sputum as well as other symptoms of heat, such as fever, thirst, yellow coating of the tongue and rapid pulse. Cough due to dryness usually occurs in the dry season and is accompanied by various dry symptoms, such as dryness of the nose, mouth and lips.

Most coughs due to internal injuries have a gradual onset and run a chronic course. They occur under the following conditions: deficiency of *yin* or *qi* of the lungs, accumulation of phlegm-damp or phlegm-heat in the lungs and attack of the lungs by liver fire. Therefore, cough may be of deficiency type or of excess type with its origin in deficiency. Although cough always indicates impairment of the lungs, pathological changes may not be confined to the lungs. Phlegm accumulated in the lungs may be produced by a hypofunctioning spleen which fails to transport all the fluid so that surplus fluid becomes phlegm or by fire attacking the lungs originating from a depressed liver. Deficiency of *yin* results in dry cough with no expectoration or scanty sputum that is difficult to expectorate. Other dryness symptoms due to *yin* deficiency may also occur, such as dryness of the mouth and lips, reddened tongue with little coating and thready, rapid pulse. In deficiency of *qi*, the cough is feeble and accompanied by shortness of breath, expectoration of thin sputum, lassitude, spontaneous sweating and susceptibility to colds. Profuse expectoration characterizes both phlegm-damp and phlegm-heat accumulation in the lungs, but the sputum is thin and whitish in the former, and sticky and yellowish in the latter.

Dyspnea. Dyspnea is either of excess type or deficiency type. Wind, cold, heat, damp and phlegm cause dyspnea of excess type. Discrimination of the pathogenic factors is based on the general conditions, accompanying symptoms and quantity and appearance of the sputum. Dyspnea of deficiency type occurs either in deficiency of lung *qi* or in failure of the kidneys to receive air. Dyspnea due to deficiency of lung *qi* is accompanied by lack of energy and strength. Dyspnea due to failure of the kidneys in receiving air is marked by prolonged exhalation which is aggravated upon exertion and accompanying symptoms showing hypofunction of the kidneys (e.g., aching of the loins, nocturia, edema of the legs).

## DIFFERENTIATION OF SYNDROMES

### I. Excess syndromes of the lungs

The lungs are delicate and vulnerable to attack by various exogenous pathogenic factors. And because the lungs are in charge of superficial body resistance, they are often the first to display symptoms when exogenous affections attack the superficial part of the body. These symptoms typically involve upper respiratory infections. If the general symptoms of a condition include marked chills and fever but the respiratory symptoms are inconspicuous, this indicates an exterior syndrome without reference to the lungs. However, if respiratory symptoms are prominent (cough, asthma, expectoration, etc.) and are combined with an exterior syndrome, this indicates a syndrome of the lungs, such as invasion of the lungs by wind-cold, wind-heat or wind-dryness. Here, the word "wind" has dual implications: it indicates the sudden onset and short duration of the illness, and it emphasizes the accompanying exterior syndrome.

If the lungs have been deeply invaded and there are no manifestations to suggest the presence of exterior syndrome (particularly chills and floating pulse), the diagnosis should be limited to the lungs with omission of the prefix "wind," e.g., affection of the lungs by heat or by dryness (or simply heat in the lungs, dryness of the lungs).

It should be emphasized that differentiating the pathogenic factors depends upon clinical manifestations rather than atmospheric changes. The clinical picture of excess syndromes of the lungs consists of general manifestations, such as fever, reddened tongue with yellow coating and rapid pulse, and specific manifestations, such as cough and expectoration. Among the specific manifestations, the character of the sputum is usually most significant.

## II. Deficiency syndromes of the lungs

The common deficiency syndromes of the lungs are deficiency of *yin* and deficiency of *qi*. Both are characterized by gradual onset and chronic course, but the former displays "dry symptoms" (dry cough or cough with scanty expectoration) and relative exuberance of *yang* or endogenous heat, while the latter manifests symptoms indicating lack of energy or strength (feeble cough, shortness of breath and lassitude). Furthermore, because deficiency of lung *qi* involves the lungs' failure in disseminating fluid, this condition causes the lungs to retain fluid which turns into phlegm and is manifested as profuse expectoration of thin sputum. However, if the expectoration is associated with anorexia, abdominal distension and loose bowels, the phlegm originates from the hypofunctioning spleen, and a diagnosis of hypofunction of both the lungs and the spleen is appropriate.

# COMMON SYNDROMES IN INTERNAL MEDICINE

**1. Deficiency of lung *qi*** (occurring in chronic bronchitis, pulmonary emphysema, pulmanory tuberculosis)

Primary manifestations: Feeble cough accompained by expectoration of thin whitish sputum, and in severe cases dyspnea or shortness of breath, pale complexion, lassitude, spontaneous sweating, pale tongue with thin whitish coating and thready, feeble pulse.

Principle of treatment: Replenish lung *qi*.

Formula of choice: Bufei Tang (Lung-invigorating Decoction).

**2. Deficiency of lung *yin*** (occurring in pulmanry tuberculosis, chronic bronchitis)

Primary manifestations: Dry cough with no sputum or scanty, sticky or blood-streaked sputum, dryness in the mouth and throat, hoarseness of voice, afternoon fever, night sweating, malar flush, heat sensation in the chest, palms and soles, dry and reddend tongue and rapid, thready pulse.

Principle of treatment: Replenish *yin* and mositen the lungs.

Formula of choice: Baihe Gujin Tang (Lily Decoction for Strengthening the Lungs).

**3. Invasion of the lungs by wind-cold** (occurring in colds, acute bronchitis, bronchial asthma)

Primary manifestations: Chilliness and mild fever, no sweating, headache, stuffy and runny nose, cough or asthma with expectoration of thin and whitish sputum, white coating of the tongue and floating, tense pulse.

Principle of treatment: Dispel wind and cold from the lungs.

Formula of choice: Xingsu San (Apricot Kernel and Perilla Powder).

**4. Invasion of the lungs by wind-heat** (occurring in influenza, acute bronchitis, bronchial asthma, early stages of general infectious diseases)

Primary manifestation: Chilliness and fever, aversion to wind, sore throat, cough or asthma with expectoration of yellow, thick sputum, yellow tongue coating and rapid, floating pulse.

Principle of treatment: Dispel wind and clear the lungs of heat.

Formula of choice: Sangju Yin (Decoction of Mulberry Leaf and Chrysanthemum).

**5. Invasion of the lungs by heat** (occurring in acute and chronic bronchitis, pneumonia, bronchial asthma)

Primary manifestation: Cough or asthma with expectoration of thick, yellow sputum, fever, thirst, concentrated urine and constipation, reddened tongue with yellow coating and rapid, slippery pulse.

Principle of treatment: Clear the lungs of heat.

Formula of choice: Ma Xing Shi Gan Tang (Decoction of Ephedra, Apricot Kernel, Gypsum and Liquorice).

**6. Invasion of the lungs by dryness** (occurring in colds and bronchitis)

Primary manifestations: Dry cough or cough accompanied by scanty, sticky sputum difficult to expectorate, dry nose and throat, reddened tip and thin yellow coating of the tongue and rapid pulse.

Principle of treatment: Relieve the dryness of the lungs.

Formula of choice: Sang Xing Tang (Decoction of Mulberry Leaf and Apricot Kernel).

**7. Accumulation of phlegm-damp in the lungs** (occurring in asthmatic bronchitis, bronchiectasis)

Primary manifestations: Productive cough or asthma with copious expectoroation of white and frothy or glutinous sputum, feeling of fullness in the chest, rattling sounds of sputum in the throat, greasy, white tongue coating and soft, slippery pulse.

Principle of treatment: Remove damp and phlegm.

Formula of choice: Erchen Tang (Decoction of Two Old Drugs).

**8. Accumulation of phlegm-heat in the lungs** (occurring in acute bronchitis, chronic bronchitis with acute exacerbation, bronchiectasis with secondary infection, pneumonia, bronchial asthma or pulmonary emphysema complicated by infection)

Primary manifestations: Cough accompanied by dyspnea and expectoration of copious yellow, thick or purulent sputum, fever, thirst, chest pain, concentrated urine, constipation, reddened tongue with yellow, greasy coating and rapid, slippery pulse.

Principle of treatment: Clear the lungs of heat and phlegm.

Formula of choice: Qingqi Huatan Wan (Bolus for Clearing Heat and Phlegm).

**9. Attack of the lungs by liver fire:** See section titled Common Syndrome Involving Two Viscera.

## Section 5    SYNDROMES OF THE KIDNEYS AND URINARY BLADDER

The kidneys store vital essence, take charge of reproduction, growth and development, regulate water circulation, help the lungs receive air (inhale), supply the bones with marrow and determine the condition of the bones. Most kidney diseases involve deficiency.

The urinary bladder and the kidneys are closely related, both anatomically and functionally. The kidneys control the urinary bladder's storing and discharging of urine.

## SYMPTOMS AND SIGNS

The vital essence stored in the kidneys (the chief constituent of kidney *yin*) is the basis of reproduction, growth and development, the formation of marrow, the nourishment of the bones and the replenishment of the brain. If the vital essence in the kidneys is insufficient, the symptoms outlined in Talbe VI-III may occur.

**Table VI-III. Symptoms Resulting from Insufficient Vital Essence in the Kidneys**

|  | In Children | In Adults |
|---|---|---|
| Impairment of: |  |  |
| Growth and development | Retardation of growth | Premature senility |
| Reproduction | Delayed maturity | Sterility |
| Brain | Underdevelopment of mental faculties | Slow reactions, dizziness, tinnitus, hypomnesia |
| Bones | Delayed closure of fontanel, rickets | Softening of the bones, weakness of the legs |
| Teeth | Retarded eruption | Luxation of the teeth |

Kidney *yang* warms the body, heats up the spleen to assist in food digestion, helps the lungs receive air, regulates water metabolism, assists the urinary bladder in storing and discharging urine and acts as the dynamic force behind reproduction (sexual potency). Symptoms associated with deficiency of kidney *yang* are summarized in Table VI-IV.

**Table VI-IV. Symptoms Resulting from Deficiency of Kidney *Yang***

|  | Symptoms |
|---|---|
| Insufficiecy of: |  |
| Warming the body | Chilliness, intolerance to cold, cold limbs |
| Heating up the spleen | Diarrhea with fluid stools containing undigested food or diarrhea occurring before dawn daily |
| Helping the lungs receive air | Dyspnea or asthma |
| Regulating water metabolism | Oliguria, edema |
| Assisting the urinary bladder | Dysuria, incontinence of urine |
| Dynamic force behind reproduction | Impotence, hyposexuality |

Diseases of the kidneys involve another typical symptom which is related to patho-anatomy rather than pathophysiology, namely pain in the lumbar regions.

A diseased urinary bladder causes abnormal changes in the urine and disturbs urination. However, urination disturbances in chronic cases are often attributed to hypofunction of the kidneys.

Following is a detailed discussion of symptoms commonly seen in kidney and urinary bladder diseases.

Lumbago. Ailments of the kidneys often cause pain in the lumbar region. Exogenous pathogenic factors (such as cold-damp or damp-heat) attacking meridians and collaterals or stagnated *qi* and blood due to muscle strain or traumatic injuries cause lumbago of excess type. In these cases, the practitioner must tonify the kidneys as well as remove cold-damp, damp-heat or blood stasis. If cold-damp causes the lumbago, it will manifest itself as pain characterized by an association with cold sensations. It will be aggravated by cold, damp weather. A heat sensation in the lumbar regions accompanies lumbago due to damp-heat. If blood stasis causes the lumbago, it is usually accompanied by a history of trauma, and the pain is characterized by fixed location, difficulty in turning over and local tenderness. Examining the tongue is an important element in diagnosis. It will have a white, greasy coating in lumbago due to cold-damp, a yellow, greasy coating in lumbago due to damp-heat, and the tongue will be purplish in lumbago due to blood stasis. Lumbago of deficiency type is accompanied by weakness of the loins and legs which is aggravated by physical exertion and alleviated by bed rest.

Seminal emissions. Both types of involuntary discharge of semen — nocturnal emissions as a result of lustful dreams and spontaneous emissions which occur during sleep without dreams and even when the patient is awake — are related to disorders of the kidneys. Nocturnal emissions may also involve the heart and are due to deficiency of *yin* of the heart and kidneys with exuberant fire. Symptoms include excessive sexual desire, premature ejaculation and insomnia. On the other hand, spontaneous emissions result from a deficiency symdrome of the kidneys alone. Symptoms include lassitude, aching of the loins, dizziness, tinnitus and aversion to cold with cold limbs. In some cases, seminal emissions due to accumulation of damp-heat cause heat sensation in the urethra during micturition, bitterness in the mouth and a yellow, greasy tongue coating.

Impotence. In a majority of cases, impotence is a symptom of deficiency of kidney *yang* due to overindulgence in sex. Impotence caused by a downward drive of damp-heat is also common. In addition, anxiety impairing the heart and spleen and fright impairing the kidneys may also lead to impotence. Therefore, a detailed patient history is required for proper diagnosis. The physician should also watch for these accompanying symptoms: pallor, listlessness, weakness of the loins and legs and general aversion to cold in deficiency of kidney *yang*; yellow, greasy tongue coating and soft, rapid pulse in the presence of damp-heat; insomnia and anorexia when the heart and spleen are impaired.

Edema. According to traditional medical theory, the lungs, spleen and kidneys regulate water metabolism. Therefore, edema may be attributed to the functional disturbance of any of these visceral organs.

(1) Edema due to impaired function of the lungs: Exogenous pathogenic factors, particularly "wind," may attack the lungs and impair their ability to regulate the water passages. This may lead to edema called "wind-edema." The prodromal syndrome wind

affection (upper respiratory infection) often precedes it with symptoms including fever, aversion to wind and cold, headache, cough, sore throat and floating pulse. Usually, the edema has an acute onset, first appearing in the eyelids and face, then extending downwards.

(2) Edema due to deficiency of spleen *yang*: The transportation function of the spleen includes promoting water metabolism. If the spleen is impaired, edema which is often more marked in the limbs than other parts of the body may occur accompanied by anorexia, abdominal distension, oliguria, loose stools, cold limbs, sallow complexion and white, slippery tongue coating.

(3) Edema due to deficiency of kidney *yang*: Among the visceral organs, the kidneys are the chief regulators of water metabolism. Deficiency of kidney *yang* may cause edema which is more marked in the lower part of the body and is accompanied by lumbago, oliguria, aversion to cold, cold limbs, pallor and whitish, moist tongue coating.

Dysuria. Acute dysuria is due to accumulation of damp-heat in the urinary bladder. It is characterized by urodynia, unduly frequent passage of urine and urgency of urination. In some cases, sudden interruptions during voiding may occur, or calculi may appear in the urine. A discharge of turbid or bloody urine may also be present.

In chronic cases, however, difficulty in urination is mostly of the deficiency type, in which urodynia is usually absent and the urine is no longer turbid. This is often attributed to a deficiency state of the kidneys but may also result from a deficiency state of the spleen occurring as a symptom of sinking spleen *qi*. Hematuria may be present if an exuberant fire secondary to a deficiency of kidney *yin* injures the blood vessels.

# DIFFERENTIATION OF SYNDROMES

## I. Syndromes of deficiency of kidney *yin*

The chief constituent of kidney *yin* is the vital essence stored in the kidneys. When it is deficient, the clinical manifestations listed in Table VI-III occur. Because of the reciprocal relationship between *yin* and *yang*, deficiency of kidney *yin* typically results in exuberance of kidney *yang* or endogenous heat. Therefore, hyperactivity of kidney *yang* may cause nocturnal emissions while endogenous heat may cause afternoon fever, malar flush and feverishness in the palms and soles.

## II. Syndromes of deficiency of kidney *yang*

Kidney *yang* performs multiple functions, including warming up the body and various visceral organs. When kidney *yang* is insufficient, "cold manifestations," such as chilliness, aversion to cold, cold limbs, pallor and pale tongue, often occur. When general cold manifestations appear with symptoms indicating involvement of the kidneys, such as aching and weakness of the loins and legs or hyposexuality, a simple diagnosis of "deficiency of kidney *yang*" can be made. However, if other functions are markedly impaired, the physician should specify the chief disorder in the diagnosis, e.g., failure of the kidneys in receiving air, hypofunction of the kidneys with edema or hypofunction of the kidneys with diarrhea.

Kidney *yang* also heats up various visceral organs to invigorate their functions. Sometimes, it may be difficult to differentiate whether diminished functional activity is confined to the kidneys or involves another visceral organ. For instance, in hypofunction of the kidneys with diarrhea, deficiency of kidney *yang*, strictly speaking, impairs the spleen. If only loose bowel movements occur before dawn daily, the diagnosis of hypofunction of the kidneys with diarrhea is adequate; but if other symptoms indicate hypofunction of the spleen, the practitioner should diagnose the condition as hypofunction of both the spleen and the kidneys or deficiency of both spleen and kidney *yang*. It is also necessary to differentiate between edema due to hypofunction of the kidneys and edema due to hypofunction of both the spleen and the kidneys.

# COMMON SYNDROMES IN INTERNAL MEDICINE

**1. Deficiency of kidney *yin*** (occurring in debility after a protracted disease, tuberculosis, diabetes mellitus, chronic nephritis, sexual neurosis, sterility)

Primary manifestations: Dizziness, forgetfulness, aching of the loins and knees, tinnitus, impaired hearing, dryness in the mouth and throat, seminal emissions, oligospermia and sterility in males and amenorrhea and infertility in females, afternoon fever, malar flush, night sweating, reddened tongue with scanty or no coating and deep and thready pulse.

Principle of treatment: Nourish kidney *yin*.

Formula of choice: Liuwei Dihuang Wan (Bolus of Six Ingredients Including Rehmannia).

**2. Deficeincy of kidney *yang* or hypofunction of the kidneys** (occurring in debility after a protracted disease, general weakness in the aged, chronic nephritis, adrenocortical insufficiency, hypothyroidism, neurasthenia)

Primary manifestations: Aching of the back and loins, chilliness, intolerance to cold, cold limbs, hyposexuality, impotence, premature ejaculation, oliguria and edema, chronic diarrhea, pallor, pale, plump tongue with thin, whitish coating and deep and thready pulse.

Principle of treatment: Warm and tonify kidney *yang*.

Formula of choice: Shenqi Wan (Bolus for Tonifying Kidney *Qi*).

**3. Deficiency of kidney *yang* with water in flood or hypofunction of the kidneys with edema** (occurring in nephrotic syndrome, heart failure)

Primary manifestations: Deficiency of kidney *yang* plus oliguria, edema, even anasarca and ascites, or cardiac palpitations and orthopnea.

Principle of treatment: Warm the kidneys and induce diuresis.

Formula of choice: Jisheng Shenqi Wan (Life-preserving Pill for Invigorating the Kidneys).

**4. Deficiency of kidney *yang* with diarrhea or hypofunction of the kidneys with diarrhea** (occurring in chronic colitis and chronic dysentery)

Primary manifestations: Deficiency of kidney *yang* plus chronic diarrhea, particularly diarrhea daily before dawn that is aggravated after exposure of the abdomen to cold.

Principle of treatment: Relieve the diarrhea by warming the kidneys.

Formula of choice: Sishen Wan (Pill of Four Miraculous Drugs).

**5. Failure of the kidneys in receiving air or assisting the lungs in receiving air** (occurring in pulmonary emphysema, cor pulmonale debility states with shortness of breath)

Primary manifestations: Deficiency of kidney *yang* plus dyspnea with prolonged exhalation, aggravated on exertion.

Principle of treatment: Tonify the kidneys to facilitate respiration.

Formula of choice: Duqi Wan (Dyspnea-relieving Pill), i.e., Liuwei Dihuang Wan (Bolus of Six Ingredients Including Rehmannia) plus *Fructus Schisandrae* (schisandra fruit).

**6. Failure of the kidneys in controlling discharge of urine or sperm** (occurring in incontinence of urine, enuresis, diabetes insipitus, chronic nephritis with nocturia, sexual disorders)

Primary manifestations: General manifestations of deficiency of the kidneys plus frequent micturition, nocturnal polyruea, dribbling of urine after voiding, incontinence of urine or enuresis, premature ejaculation and spermatorrhea.

Principle of treatment: Consolidate kidney *qi*.

Formula of choice: For failure of the kidneys in controlling urination, Suoquan Wan (Pill for Reducing Urination); for failure of the kidneys in controlling seminal discharge, Jinsuo Gujing Wan (Golden Lock Pill for Keeping the Kidney Essence).

**7. Damp-heat in the urinary bladder** (occurring in urinary infections, urolithiasis, prostatitis)

Primary manifestations: Frequency and urgency of urination, urodynia with burning sensation in the urethra or difficulty in urination, turbid or bloody urine or passage of calculi with urination, distress in the lower abdomen, yellow and greasy tongue coating and slippery and rapid pulse.

Principle of treatment: Remove damp-heat from the urinary bladder.

Formula of choice: Bazheng San (All-orientation Health-restoring Powder).

## Section 6   SYNDROMES INVOLVING TWO VISCERA (*ZANG*-ORGANS)

According to traditional medical theory, all visceral organs are related physiologically and pathologically. A diseased viscus is likely to affect other viscera, and numerous syndromes involve two or more viscera.

A syndrome involving two or more viscera has complicated manifestations consisting of some combination of the symptoms associated with the simple syndromes of the viscera involoved. For example, if a patient suffers from chronic cough, shortness of breath, cardiac palpitations aggravated during physical exertion, pale complexion, pale tongue and thready, feeble pulse, the diagnosis is deficiency of *qi* of the heart and lungs. Chronic cough often leads to deficiency of lung *qi*; shortness of breath indicates that the *qi* is already insufficient. Cardiac palpitations are a common symptom indicating impairment of the heart. Therefore, deficiency of *qi* of the heart and the lungs is a combined syndrome of deficiency of heart *qi* and deficiency of lung *qi*. It is important to determine which syndrome is the primary one and which the secondary one. If the patient's cough had existed for many years and then cardiac palpitations occurred, this would indicate that deficiency of lung *qi* had led to deficiency of heart *qi*. If cardiac palpitations had preceded the cough, this would indicate that deficiency of heart *qi* had led to deficiency of lung *qi*.

The following syndromes involving two viscera are commonly encountered in internal medicine.

**1. Deficiency of *yin* of the liver and kidneys** (occurring in anemia, hypertension, chronic hepatitis, neurosis, Meniere's syndrome, menstrual disorders)

Primary manifestations: Dizziness, tinnitus, blurred vision, irritability, irascibility, aching and weakness of the loins and legs, feverishness in the palms and soles or numbness of the limbs and muscle twitching, seminal emissions in men and oligomenorrhea or amenorrhea in women, reddened tongue with scanty coating and thready, taut pulse.

Principle of treatment: Nourish the liver and the kidneys.

Formula of choice: Qiju Dihuang Wan (Bolus of Rehmannia with Wolfberry and Chrysanthemum).

**2. Incoordination between the liver and spleen and/or the stomach** (occurring in peptic ulcer, chronic gastritis, hepatitis, other digestive diseases)

Primary manifestations: Symptoms indicating stagnation of liver *qi* together with weakness of the spleen and/or the stomach including irascibility, hypochondriac pain, loss of appetite, abdominal distension, borborygmi, loose bowels, feeling of stuffiness and pain in the epigastrium, belching, acid regurgitation, nausea, vomiting, whitish, greasy tongue coating and taut pulse.

Principle of treatment: Soothe the liver and regulate the spleen and/or the stomach.

Formula of choice: Xiaoyao San (Ease Powder).

**3. Deficiency of *qi* and blood in the heart and spleen** (occurring in neurosis, anemia)

Primary manifestations: Cardiac palpitations and fidgetiness, insomnia, dream-disturbed sleep, forgetfulness, anorexia, abdominal distension, loose bowels, lassitude, lack of strength, sallow complexion, whitish tongue coating and thready pulse.

Principle of treatment: Replenish the heart and spleen.

Formula of choice: Guipi Tang (Decoction for Restoration of the Spleen).

**4. Incoordination between the heart and kidneys** (occurring in neurosis, anemia, other chronic consumptive diseases)

Primary manifestations: Aching of the loins and weakness of the legs, dizziness, tinnitus, insomnia, hypomnesis, cardiac palpitations and fidgetiness, nocturnal emissions, night sweating, reddened tongue with little coating and thready, rapid pulse.

Principle of treatment: Restore coordination between the heart and the kidneys.

Formula of choice: Liuwei Dihuang Wan (Bolus of Six Ingredients Including Rehmannia) plus Jiaotai Wan (Coordinating Pill).

**5. Deficiency of *yang* of the spleen and kidneys** (occurring in chronic colitis, tuberculosis of the intestines, ulcerative colitis, nephrotic syndrome, liver cirrhosis with ascites)

Primary manifestations: Aversion to cold with cold extremities, lassitude, lack of strength, fatigability intractable diarrhea with stools containing undigested food or diarrhea before dawn daily, anorexia, abdominal distension or oliguria and edema, pale complexion, pale, plump tongue with whitish, thin or whitish, greasy coating and teeth prints at its borders.

Principle of treatment: Warm and tonifty the spleen and kidneys.

Formula of choice: For chronic diarrhea, Fuzi Lizhong Tang (Decoction for Regulating Middle-*jiao* with Aconite) plus Sishen Wan (Pill of Four Miraculous Drugs); for edema, Zhenwu Tang (Decoction for Invigorating *Yang*) plus Wuling San (Five Drugs Powder).

**6. Deficiency of *qi* of the lungs and spleen** (occurring in chronic bronchitis, pulmonary emphysema)

Primary manifestations: Chronic cough, profuse expectoration of thin, frothy sputum, loss of appetite, abdominal distension, loose bowels, lassitude, fatigability, edema (in some cases), pale tongue with whitish coating and thready, feeble pulse.

Principle of treatment: Tonify the lungs and spleen.

Formula of choice: Liu Junzi Tang (Decoction of Six Ingredients).

**7. Deficiency of *yin* of the lungs and kidneys** (occurring in pulmonary tuberculosis, other consumptive diseases)

Primary manifestations: Cough with scanty expectoration or hemoptysis, emaciation, aching and weakness of the loins and legs, hectic fever, malar flush, night sweating, dryness of the throat and mouth, seminal emissions, reddened tongue with little coating and thready, rapid pulse.

Principle of treatment: Replenish the lungs and kidneys.

Formula of choice: Maiwei Dihuang Wan (Bolus of Rehmannia plus Ophiopogon and Schisandra).

# PART TWO

# CHAPTER VII   COMMON COLD

Among viral infections of the upper respiratory tract, the most common one is the cold. Rhinoviruses cause most colds. Droplets from the nasopharynx provide the main route of infection. Immunity after a cold is very transient because a common immunizing antigen is often lacking, the site of the infection is localized and there is an absence of viremia. Consequently, many individuals have more than one cold a year.

Although colds have few sequelae and cause practically no deaths, their frequent occurrence causes considerable discomfort and thus significant economic loss for the community. No specific therapy or immunization is available at present. The prospects for finding a vaccine are poor because there are many strains of rhinoviruses, which may cause the common cold, and because the immunity lasts only a short time (it appears dependent on local mechanisms). Thus, traditional theories and practices for preventing and treating colds are still relevant.

Traditional Chinese medicine holds that an attack of pathogenic "wind" causes the common cold. Thus, the Chinese people popularly describe coming down with a cold as "catching wind." Symptoms include stuffy and runny nose, sneezing, sore throat and hoarseness of voice. General symptoms, such as chilliness, fever, headache and aching all over the body may appear, but they are often mild or absent. Colds usually last for three to seven days and patients recover without complications.

## ETIOLOGY AND PATHOGENESIS

Pathogenic wind is the predominant etiological factor in colds. It invades the upper respiratory tract and the body surface when body resistance is low, which typically occurs when there is a sudden climatic change. The pathogenic wind combines with cold in winter, heat in spring and damp-heat in summer, taking advantage of untimely climatic changes to attack the body.

The attack on the body is closely related to body resistance, so if one's vital energy is low due to an irregular life style, drenching by rain, negligence regarding changes in temperature or overfatigue, the likelihood of invasion increases. A patient with chronic bronchitis or bronchiectasis is also vulnerable. Furthermore, the body's constitution plays a role in the affection. A person with a *yang* deficiency is susceptible to wind-cold, and one with a *yin* deficiency is susceptible to wind-heat.

Because pathogenic wind invades through the upper respiratory tract and the body surface, pathological changes are confined to these portions of the body. (The respiratory tract and the body surface are closely related in function.) When pathogenic factors obstruct the upper respiratory tract, respiratory symptoms occur, such as cough and stuffy nose. The confrontation between the body's resistance and pathogenic factors at the superficial portion of the body results in chilliness and fever.

# DIAGNOSIS OF SYNDROMES

Colds typically begin with a stuffy and runny nose, sneezing, hoarseness of voice and sometimes headache and chilliness. Then, fever, cough and itching or pain of the throat occur.

The following points are significant to the traditional diagnosis of colds:

1. Differentiation of cold and heat syndromes. Generally speaking, wind-cold affections are characterized by marked chilliness, mild fever and stuffy nose with thin mucous secretion, while wind-heat affections are characterized by fever with mild chilliness and sore throat with local redness and swelling. Sometimes a wind-cold syndrome may turn into a wind-heat syndrome, marked by sore throat and mucopurulent nasal discharge — an example of transformation of cold into heat.

2. Recognition of combined pathogenic factors. If the pathogenic wind invades the human body in combination with damp as often occurs during rainy seasons, the patient usually experiences a headache which feels as though the head were tightly bound, accompanied by fullness in the chest and nausea. Combination with summer-heat is characterized by fever, sweating, thirst, scanty concentrated urine and yellow, greasy tongue coating.

3. Determination of deficiency or excess type. The common cold is of excess type in most cases. However, a deficiency syndrome characterized by spontaneous sweating and aversion to wind may be present. Patients in a deficiency state often suffer from repeated colds.

Clinical manifestations of syndromes occurring in the common cold:

1. Exterior syndrome of cold (Syndrome of wind-cold). Chilliness and mild fever with no sweating or thirst, general aching, stuffy and runny nose, sneezing, itching of the throat, cough with thin expectoration or dry cough, thin and white tongue coating and floating, tense pulse.

Exterior syndrome of cold-damp (Syndrome of wind-cold combined with damp). In addition to the above symptoms, this syndrome includes persistent low fever, headache as if the head were tightly bound, heaviness of the limbs or fullness in the chest, nausea, anorexia and greasy tongue coating.

2. Exterior syndrome of heat (Syndrome of wind-heat). Fever with mild chilliness, sweating, thirst, headache, redness and pain of the throat, cough with mucopurulent expectoration, thin and yellowish tongue coating and floating, rapid pulse.

Exterior syndrome of heat-damp (Syndrome of wind-heat combined with damp). In addition to the above symptoms, this syndrome includes persistent fever in spite of sweating, fidgets, concentrated urine, nausea, anorexia and yellowish, greasy tongue coating.

3. Exterior syndrome of deficiency. Here, deficiency chiefly refers to deficiency of *qi*, especially the superficial defensive power. Symptoms include repeated attacks of chilliness with mild fever, spontaneous sweating, headache, stuffy nose, cough with thin

mucous expectoration, feeble voice, shortness of breath, lassitude, white tongue coating and floating, weak pulse.

## TREATMENT

### 1. Exterior syndrome of cold

Herbal medication: Relieve the exterior syndrome with drugs pungent in flavor and warm in property. The following prescriptions are recommended:

(1) Decoction of green onion and fresh ginger — Boil 3-7 pieces of the white part of green onions and 3-5 slices of fresh ginger with an appropriate quantity of sugar added, to be taken while hot. This is a simple and popular decoction for preventing colds after being drenched by rain or being exposed to cold. It can also be used for treating mild colds which involve exterior cold syndromes at the outset.

(2) Antiphlogistic Powder of Schizonepeta and Ledebouriella (Jin Fang Baidu San) — Indicated in both the exterior syndrome of cold and exterior syndrome of cold-damp. If the damp syndrome is marked, Herba Agastachis and Cortex Magnolia Officinalis may be added.

Acupuncture: Needling at Fengchi (GB 20), Lieque (L 7), Fengmen (BL 12) and Hegu (LI 4) points.

### 2. Exterior syndrome of heat

Herbal medication: Relieve the exterior syndrome with drugs pungent in flavour and cool in property.

(1) Powder of Lonicera and Forsythia (Yin Qiao San) — Make into decoction for treating exterior syndrome of heat. Pill and tablet preparations are also available called Antiphlogistic Pill (or Tablet) of Lonicera and Forsythia (Yin Qiao Jiedu Wan [Pian]). The dosage of the latter is 2 pills (or 8 tablets) twice a day. The composition of the pill or tablet is generally the same as that of the powder but with some minor modifications.

(2) Antipyretic Granules for Colds (Ganmao Tuire Chongji) — A new preparation for treating colds with exterior heat syndrome. Dosage is 2-3 packs 2-3 times a day taken in hot water.

(3) Powder of Agastachis for Restoring Health (Huoxiang Zhengqi San) — Make into decoction for treating exterior syndrome of heat combined with damp. Tablet and extract preparations are also available, but this medication is usually indicated in mild cases.

Acupuncture: Needling at Dazhui (GV 14), Quchi (LI 11), Hegu (LI 4), Chize (LU 5) and Waiguan (TE 5) points.

### 3. Exterior syndrome of deficiency

Herbal medication: Relieve the exterior syndrome with appropriate drugs and at the same time reinforce *qi* with tonics.

(1) Ginseng and Perilla Drink (Shen Su Yin) — Make into decoction for treating exterior syndrome of deficiency.

(2) Jade-screen Powder (Yupingfeng San) — A decoction made of this powder and administered in small daily dosages over a long period of time can prevent the recurrence of colds in patients with weakened defensive power against changes of weather.

Moxibustion: Apply moxa stick to Zusanli (ST 36) and Shimen (CV 5) points to prevent the recurrence of colds.

## MODERN RESEARCH

It is difficult to evaluate a therapy for the treatment of a self-limited disease like the common cold. However, controlled studies have shown that traditional therapy shortened the course of the disease and relieved the symptoms quickly. Traditional therapy has several other advantages. It relieves symptoms without side effects when administered properly, because the treatment is based on the individual patient's condition and applied differently to different patients. Chilliness and fever, once relieved, seldom recur, probably because of the anti-viral effect of some ingredients contained in *Radix Ledebouriellae*, *Flos Lonicerae* and *Radix Isatidis*, and because these herbs promote the body's ability to resist disease by regulating the *yin-yang* balance. Research has also shown that *Radix Astragali*, the main ingredient of Jade-screen Powder, promotes the blood interferon level induced by virus. This preventive effect, also shown in a double-blind controlled test, is of particular interest in treating individuals vuluerable to recurrent colds.

# CHAPTER VIII   CHRONIC BRONCHITIS

Chronic bronchitis causes increased mucous secretion in the tracheobronchial tract, resulting in a productive cough which is present on most days for a minimum of three months of the year and for at least two consecutive years. It is the most common debilitating respiratory disease in China as well as in other countries, particularly among the aged.

Its cause is not yet clear, but several factors are strongly associated with this disease. Cigarette smoking has been shown to be the most important predisposing factor. Some authors hold that pneumococci and Haemophilus influenzae organisms cause infections that result in chronic bronchitis. However, others believe that the infections are the result rather than the cause of this chronic disease. Endogenous factors may also be involved. A genetic abnormality that affects mucus production may impair bronchial clearance and harm protective mechanisms, leading to recurrent or chronic infection. Bronchial allergies may increase secretion of mucus or cause one to be more susceptible to bronchial infection. Exposure to cold exacerbates the condition and may also be related to constitutional hypersensitivity.

Goblet cells in the epithelial lining and bronchial mucous glands lying beneath the epithelium produce the secretion of the tracheobronchial trees. In chronic bronchitis, the mucous glands increase in thickness, and goblet cells increase in number. These changes, along with an increase in the volume of tracheobronchial secretions, explain the chronic productive cough. But late in the course of chronic bronchitis, severe airway obstruction usually occurs, and this cannot be entirely explained by the narrowing of central airways caused by mucous gland thickening and obstruction by the secretions themselves. Small airway obstruction resulting from goblet cell proliferation or bronchiolitis may play an important role. Other morphologic changes accompanying goblet cell and bronchial gland abnormalities include fragmentation of the mucosa, destruction of cilia, inflammatory cell infiltration of the epithelium and subepithelium and basal cell hyperplasia and squamous metaplasia of columnar epithelium. Once ciliated mucosae have been disrupted, airway defenses become more susceptible to subsequent injury.

Owing to the complexity of its pathogenesis and pathological changes, chronic bronchitis is difficult to treat, especially where a long-term cure is concerned. Western medicine routinely uses bronchodilators, mucolytics and expectorants. The benefits of these agents are chiefly symptomatic — none can reverse the pathological changes or improve the patient's constitution and resistance to bronchial infection. Use of antibiotics is only rational for the treatment and prophylaxis of acute purulent exacerbations. Administering corticosteroids has limited effectiveness in treating chronic bronchitis, and the undesirable side effects of long-term corticosteriod therapy may outweigh the benefits. Hence, the search for effective herbal drugs is justified.

In traditional Chinese medicine, chronic bronchitis is closely linked to "cough," "phlegm" and "dyspnea" in syndrome diagnosis and treatment.

## ETIOLOGY AND PATHOGENESIS

The hallmarks of chronic bronchitis are a chronic cough and sputum production. Shortness of breath may later become prominent. From the traditional point of view, cough is a common symptom of lung disease, but the production of sputum is not necessarily confined to disorders of the lungs. Purulent sputum usually results when exogenous pathogenic factors, particularly heat, attack the lungs. Production of nonpurulent voluminous phlegm is often attributed to dysfunction of the spleen. In this case, the lungs merely store the phlegm and cough it up. Accumulation of phlegm in the lungs renders them vulnerable to repeated attacks by exogenous pathogenic factors, resulting in acute exacerbations. Shortness of breath with difficulty in exhalation, usually occurring late in the course of chronic bronchitis indicates that the kidneys are involved, since they help the lungs respire, and protracted difficulty in respiration with prolonged exhalation is characteristic of impaired kidneys.

In summary, traditional Chinese medicine considers chronic bronchitis a disease of the lungs that also involves impairment of the functions of the spleen and the kidneys. Only during acute exacerbations do exogenous pathogens play an important role.

## DIFFERENTIAL DIAGNOSIS OF SYNDROMES

Chronic bronchitis appears as several main syndrome patterns. An individual patient may suffer from one or more syndromes at a time, and the syndrome may change from one to another in the same patient at different stages in the course of the disease.

## DEFICIENCY SYNDROMES

Most chronic bronchitis patients are in a deficiency state of the lungs, spleen or kidneys.

1. Deficiency of the lungs: Characterized by frequent cough and expectoration. The patient may have spontaneous sweating, usually feels an aversion to draughts and is prone to catching colds. The tongue is often pale with whitish coating, and the pulse is weak.

2. Deficiency of the spleen: Characterized by profuse production of phlegm. Besides exhibiting respiratory symptoms, patients often complain of loss of appetite, abdominal distension and loose stools. The tongue coating is often whitish and greasy, and the pulse is slippery.

3. Deficiency of the kidneys: Characterized by shortness of breath with prolonged expiration accompanied by coughing and expectoration. The patient may feel an aversion to cold with cold extremities, soreness in the loins, limpness in the legs and nocturia. The pulse is thready and weak, especially at the cubit.

## EXCESS SYNDROMES

Chronic bronchitis sufferers usually experience excess syndromes during acute exacerbations.

1. Acute exacerbation of the cold type: Usually precipitated by catching a cold and manifested by an aggravated cough and expectoration of voluminous thin sputum, whitish in color. The pulse is often floating and tense.

2. Acute exacerbation of the heat type: Characterized by purulent sputum and may be accompanied by fever, dryness of the mouth, concentrated urine and constipation. The tongue coating is usually yellow, the pulse rapid and slippery.

## TREATMENT

The general rule of herbal treatment for chronic bronchitis is to invigorate or reinforce the function of the lungs, spleen and/or kidneys. However, if acute exacerbation exists, priority should be given to removing the pathogenic factors.

## ACUTE EXACERBATIONS

1. Acute exacerbation of the cold type: Use Xiaoqinglong Tang (Minor Decoction of Blue Dragon; see Appendix for composition). In this formula, *Herba Ephedrae* (ephedra), *Ramulus Cinnamomi* (cinnamom twigs), *Herba Asari* (asarum herb) and *Rhizoma Zingiberis* (dried ginger) combine to expel cold, mostly through diaphoresis. Modern research has shown, however, that *Herba Ephedrae* not only causes diaphoresis but also has bronchodilatory, anti-inflammatory, anti-allergic, anti-pyretic and anti-viral actions. Apparently, these actions help control an acute exacerbation, whether it was caused by an upper respiratory viral infection or by an allergic mechanism related to exposure to cold or allergens. *Radix Cinnamomi* can cause dilatation of the peripheral blood vessels and has antibacterial (e.g., anti-pneumococcic) and anti-viral (e.g., anti-influenzal) actions. *Rhizoma Zingiberis* is also a vasodilator. *Herba Asari* is both an antipyretic and an analgesic.

*Rhizoma Pinelliae Praeparata* (pinellia tuber) is another important ingredient in this formula. It is a phlegm-resolving drug indicated for treating excessive thin sputum but not for purulent viscid sputum. Modern research has shown that it can inhibit the secretion induced by pilocarpine. Therefore, it is not an expectorant in the Western medical sense.

2. Acute exacerbation of the heat type: The formulae used for this acute exacerbation are very different from the formula mentioned above. Qingjin Huatan Tang (Decoction for Clearing the Lungs and Resolving Phlegm) is an example (see Appendix for composition). Compared with Xiaoqinglong Tang, this formula has more ingredients with broad antibacterial actions, such as *Radix Scutellariae* (scutellaria root), *Fructus Gardeniae* (capejasmine fruit), *Radix Ophiopogonis* (ophiopogon root) and *Rhizoma Anemarrhenae* (anemarrhena rhizoma), and more potent antipyretic ingredients, such as *Radix Scutellariae*, *Radix Platycodi* (platycodon root) and *Rhizoma Anemarrhenae*. The phlegm-resolving ingredients contained in this formaula, such as *Radix Platycodi* and

*Bulbus Fritillariae Cirrhosae* (tendrilled fritillary bulb) also differ from *Rhizoma Pinelliae Praeparata*. They are expectorants that increase and liquefy bronchial secretions, thus making the phlegm easier for the patient to cough up and spit out.

## DEFICIENCY SYNDROMES

1. Deficiency of the lungs: Tonify the lungs and relieve cough with Bufei Tang (Lung-tonifying Decoction), in which *Radix Ginseng* (ginseng) and *Radix Astragali* (astragalus root) are the main tonics.

2. Deficiency of the spleen: Tonify the spleen and eliminate phlegm with Erchen Tang (Decoction of Two Old Drugs).

3. Deficiency of the kidneys: Tonify the kidneys and relieve dyspnea with Duqi Wan (Dyspnea-relieving Pill), composed of Liuwei Dihuang Wan (Bolus of Six Ingredients Including Rehmannia), a common formula for tonifying the kidney, and *Fructus Schisandrae* (schisandra fruit), an ingredient for relieving cough and dyspnea. If marked cold symptoms are present, such as aversion to cold and cold extremities, *Radix Aconiti Praeparata* (prepared aconite root) and *Cortex Cinnamomi* (cinnamon bark) are added.

Theoretically, deficiency syndromes occurring in chronic bronchitis can be divided into the above three categories, and in the course of the disease, first the lungs are involved, then the spleen and finally the kidneys. However, it is rare in clinical practice that only one of the visceral organs is involved while the others remain unaffected. Therefore, complicated prescriptions are more frequently used. Yangfei Guben Wan (Pill for Nourishing the Lungs and Strengthening the Constitution) is one example. Since the kidneys are the foundation of the inborn constitution and the spleen provides the material basis of the acquired constitution, strengthening the constitution actually refers to reinforcing the kidneys and spleen. The ingredients of the pill and their actions are listed in Table VIII-I. It is interesting to note that all the pill's major ingredients for treating chronic bronchitis without acute exacerbation are tonics which act on all three of the visceral organs.

**Table VIII-I. Actions of the Ingredients in Yangfei Guben Wan**

| Ingredients | Tonifies the lungs | Tonifies the spleen | Tonifies the kidneys |
|---|---|---|---|
| *Placenta Hominis* (human placenta) | + | | + |
| Gecko (gecko) | + | | + |
| Cordyceps (cordyceps) | + | | + |
| *Radix Ginseng* (ginseng) | + | + | |
| *Colla Cornus Cervi* (antler glue) | | | + |
| *Colla Corii Asini* (donkey-hide gelatin) | + | | |
| *Radix Glycyrrhizae* (liquorice) | + | + | |
| *Fructus Corni* (dogwood fruit) | | | + |
| *Radix Astragali* (astragalus root) | + | + | |
| *Radix Adenophorae* (adenophora root) | + | | |
| *Radix Ophiopogonis* (ophiopogon root) | + | | |
| *Herba Epimedii* (epimedium) | | | + |
| *Radix Morindae* (morinda root) | | | + |
| Poria (poria) | | + | |
| *Rhizoma Dioscoreae* (Chinese yam) | + | + | + |

# MODERN RESEARCH

In the past quarter of a century, China has done extensive research on the prevention and treatment of chronic bronchitis. Besides educating people regarding the dangers of cigarette smoking and controlling or eliminating air pollution and dusty atmospheres in workplaces, the Chinese government has focused on herbal medication research. As a result, physicians have discovered new, effective herbal drugs and applied traditional principles in new ways based on modern studies.

## DISCOVERY OF NEW, EFFECTIVE HERBAL DRUGS

In recent decades, researchers have tested hundreds of species of herbs for their effects in treating chronic bronchitis. Since the criteria for assessing effectiveness in most studies were based on the control of cough, expectoration and asthma, these new herbs are useful mainly for symptomatic relief.

*Oleum Cymopogonis*, the volatile oil of Cymbopogon distans (Nees) A. Camus (lemongrass 蕓香草 *yunxiangcao*), is a bronchodilator effective for chronic bronchitis and bronchial asthma. It is available in an aerosol spray for inhalation.

*Oleum Rhododendri Daurici*, the volatile oil of *Rhododendron dauricum L.* (dahurian rhododendron 滿山紅 *manshanhong*), is both an antitussive and an expectorant. It is available in capsules for oral administration. The usual dose for chronic bronchitis is 0.05-0.1 grams, 2-3 times daily.

*Oleum Viticis Negundo*, the volatile oil of *Vitex negundo L. var. cannabifolia* (Sieb. et Zucc.) Hand.-Mazz. (negundo chastetree 牡荆 *mujing*), is an expectorant, antitussive and antiasthmatic. It is available in capsules for oral administration. The usual dose for chronic bronchitis is 20-40 mg, 3 times daily.

*Oleum Artemisiae Lactiflorae*, the volatile oil of *Artemisia lactiflora Wall* (白花蒿 *baihuahao*), is also an expectorant and antiasthmatic, slightly more potent than *Oleum Viticis Negundo*. Its usual dose is 20 mg, 3 times a day.

## MODERN APPLICATION OF TRADITIONAL PRINCIPLES

Since chronic bronchitis results from impaired functioning of the lungs, spleen and kidneys, it is rational to seek better combinations of tonics to strengthen these organs. Scientists have developed various formulae for this purpose, most of which are modifications of traditional ones. Many have proven effective in clinical studies, and some of them have been generally accepted.

Tanyin Wan ( 痰飲丸 Pill for Treating Fluid-phlegm) is one such formula. It is composed of *Rhizoma Atractylodis* (atractylodes rhizome), *Rhizoma Atractylodis Macrocephalae* (white atractylodes rhizome), *Rhizoma Zingiberis* (dried ginger), *Radix Aconiti Lateralis Praeparata* (prepared aconite root), *Cortex Cinnamomi* (cinnamon bark), *Radix Glycyrrhizae* (liquorice), *Semen Sinapis* (mustard seed), *Fructus Perillae* (perilla seed) and *Semen Raphani* (radish seed). This formula combines two traditional prescriptions: Fugui Lizhong Tang (Decoction for Regulating the Spleen Function with Cinnamon and Aconite) and Sanzi Tang (Decoction of Three Kinds of Seeds). The former is a traditional formula for invigorating the spleen with *Radix Aconiti Lateralis Praeparata* and *Cortex Cinnamomi* for invigorating the function of the kidneys; the latter is a traditional formula for symptomatic relief of cough and expectoration.

Physicians in several cities throughout China have evaluated the efficacy of Tanyin Wan. In 1961, doctors in Xi'an reported that treatment of 195 cases of chronic bronchitis with Tanyin Wan showed an effective rate as high as 88 percent. In 1975, 97 cases of chronic bronchitis treated with this formula in Tianjin achieved an effective rate of 85.6 percent, thus confirming the earlier report from Xi'an. Also, the longer the treatment continued, the better the results. And, a majority of patients saw marked improvement in their general condition with less vulnerability to colds.

Among the three organs involved in chronic bronchitis, the kidneys seem to be the most important, especially in protracted cases with deficiency syndromes. This is because kidney deficiency usually becomes more and more pronounced as the disease develops. Researchers began to ask whether invigorating the kidney function should be the chief approach to treating chronic bronchitis. From 1972 to 1981, the ,Shanghai Medical College treated a group of 522 chronic bronchitics in eight batches. Of these patients, 64 received only antibiotics and expectorants during acute exacerbations. They were the control group. The remaining 458 patients received the same treatment during acute exacerbations, but in addition received Kidney Tonic Tablets from September to April each year to prevent the acute exacerbations that typically occur in winter. Doctors chose patients in the control group and the kidney tonic groups at random, but observed only two control groups in the first two years. The clear difference in efficacy between the control groups and the kidney tonic groups made subsequent control groups unnecessary. Of the 34 cases treated with Kidney Tonic Tablets from 1973 to 1975, 62.5 percent showed marked improvement (as shown in a five-year follow-up study) and 28.1 percent experienced a clinical cure. These results confirmed the importance of invigorating the kidney function in the treatment of chronic bronchitis.

Researchers used two kinds of Kidney Tonic Tablets in these studies. Wen Yang Pian (Kidney Tonic Tablet for Yang Deficiency), which is composed of *Radix Aconiti Lateralis Praeparata* (prepared aconite root), *Radix Rehmanniae* (rehmannia root), *Rhizoma Dioscoroeae* (Chinese yam), *Herba Epimedii* (epimedium), *Fructus Psoraleae* (psoralea fruit), *Semem Cuscutae* (dodder seed) and *Pericarpium Citri Reticulatae* (tangerine peel), is indicated for chronic bronchitis. If in the course of treatment with Wen Yang Pian thirst and constipation occur, indicating the presence of heat manifestations, Zi Yin Pian (Kidney Tonic Tablet for Yin Deficiency) should be added. It contains *Radix Rehmanniae* (rehmannia root), *Radix Asparagi* (asparagus root), *Rhizoma Dioscoreae* (Chinese yam), *Rhizoma Polygonati* (Siberian solomonseal rhizome), *Fructus Ligustri Lucidi* (lucid ligustrum fruit) and *Pericarpium Citri Reticulatae* (tangerine peel).

Another report from the China Academy of Traditional Chinese Medicine is also promising. The Academy used Guben Wan (Pill for Strengthening the Constitution) to treat chronic bronchitis with satisfactory results. This pill is composed of *Radix Astragali* (astragalus root), *Rhizoma Atractylodis Macrocephalae* (white atractylodes rhizome),

*Radix Ledebouriellae* (ledebouriella root), *Radix Codonopsis Pilosulae* (pilose asiabell root), Poria (poria), *Radix Glycyrrhizae* (liquorice), *Pericarpium Citri Reticulatae* (tangerine peel), *Rhizoma Pinelliae* (pinellia tuber), *Fructus Psoraleae* (psoralea fruit) and *Placenta Hominis* (human placenta).

Kidney Tonic Tablets chiefly contain kidney tonics, whereas Guben Wan contains spleen tonics. However, the effect of the latter was comparable to that of the former. In a long-term treatment of 140 chronic bronchitics for three-to-five years, 23 (16.4 percent) were clinically cured, 76 (54.3 percent) showed marked improvement and 26 (18.6 percent) improved, the total effective rate being 89.3 percent. In a control group in which physicians gave the patients only symptomatic treatment during acute exacerbations, 4.2 percent showed marked improvement and 33.3 percent improved, for a total effective rate of 37.5 percent.

It is interesting to note that in experimental studies both Kidney Tonic Tablets and Guben Wan, as well as Tanyin Wan, stimulate the pituitary-adrenal system and enhance the immune functions of the body. These actions may be the reason for the effect of these tonics on chronic bronchitis.

# CHAPTER IX   BRONCHIAL ASTHMA

Bronchial asthma is a disease of the airways, characterized by recurrent attacks of paroxysmal dyspnea, with wheezing and coughing caused by reversible bronchial obstruction. Early in the asthmatic attack, the spasm of the bronchial smooth muscle is the most important factor; with time, the role of inspissated mucous plugs, resulting from production of excessive mucus and swelling of the bronchial mucous membrane caused by inflammatory infiltrates, may be more important.

Most physicians believe there is a genetic basis for asthma. Many asthmatics have a predisposition to allergy. They all share a basic hyper-reactivity of the airways that makes them unusually susceptible to a great variety of substances that induce bronchospasms.

In modern medicine bronchial asthma is classified as either extrinsic or intrinsic. Extrinsic asthma usually begins during childhood. In this type of asthma, environmental allergens provoke the attack. Common allergens include pollens, animal dander, some foods (especially eggs), fish and shrimps, inert dusts, house mites and various drugs.

Intrinsic asthma usually begins during middle age. The attack is often associated with upper respiratory infection, especially viral infection. Whether this represents an allergic reaction to the infecting agent or is merely a nonspecific response of hyper-reactive bronchi to the infection is uncertain. Psychological stress, physical exertion and cold air may also induce asthma.

Asthma occurs characteristically as episodes of dyspnea with intervals of complete or nearly complete remission. At the onset of an attack, the patient experiences a sensation of suffocation and tightness in the chest, with coughing and wheezing. Then dyspnea may become severe, and loud, wheezing, prolonged expiration results, preceded by a short gasping inspiration. In a severe attack the patient is extremely dyspneic and orthopneic, and is often most comfortable sitting forward with the arms leaning on some support. There is an indrawing of the soft tissues of the neck, and the accessory muscles are active. Cyanosis is marked. The sputum is usually viscid and difficult to expectorate. A purulent appearance is commonly caused by infection. The attack often lasts from half an hour to several hours. If the attack persists for many hours or days without remission despite treatment, the patient is considered to be in "status asthmaticus," a condition often associated with signs of exhaustion.

Some patients experience a gradual change in the character of the disorder. Attacks become less frequent and less severe, but the remission is less complete. The patient develops chronic airway obstruction. This state is usually associated with chronic cough and sputum, and the patient's capacity for physical exertion progressively lessens.

## ETIOLOGY AND PATHOGENESIS

In traditional Chinese medicine, asthma is attributed to a constitutional defect that results in abnormal production of phlegm. Existence of insidious phlegm in the lungs (respiratory system) is the basic mechanism of asthma. A variety of factors, such as cold, infections, emotional distress, improper diet and physical exertion, can trigger an asthmatic episode by provoking the phlegm to obstruct the airways.

The role of phlegm is so much emphasized in the pathogenesis of asthma because the audible wheezing is believed to be produced by the phlegm in the airways. Also, remission is commonly preceded by copious expectoration and phlegm eliminating drugs are usually necessary to treat asthma.

Traditional Chinese medicine holds that although asthma is a respiratory disorder, its pathological changes are not confined to the lungs. As a constitutional disease, it involves the kidneys and the spleen, because the kidneys are the foundation of the native constitution and the spleen determines the acquired constitution. Furthermore, the kidneys aid the lungs in respiration. Diminished kidney function is marked by dyspnea with prolonged expiration. A dysfunctioning spleen produces excess phlegm. Therefore, bronchial asthma is associated with obstruction of the airways in the lungs, excessive production of phlegm by the spleen and failure of the kidneys in receiving air.

## DIFFERENTIAL DIAGNOSIS OF SYNDROMES

Diagnosis of bronchial asthma depends on the patient's history and clinical manifestations. After making the diagnosis, the physician must differentiate among syndromes in order to prescribe the correct herbal medication.

During the attack, asthma follows one of two main syndrome patterns: cold type and heat type.

1. Asthma of cold type: Dysnea with coughing and wheezing is usually preceded by sneezing, watery nasal discharge and itching of the throat. The patient may feel chilly or have an aversion to cold. The sputum is thin and frothy, the tongue coating whitish and slippery and the pulse tense and floating.

2. Asthma of heat type: The attack may be preceded by fever and cough. The patient is often irritable, has a flushed face, dire thrist and the desire for cold drink. Constipation frequently occurs. The sputum is yellowish, sticky and difficult to expectorate; the tongue is reddened with a yellowish, greasy coating; the pulse is slippery and rapid.

Traditional medicine's classification of asthmatic attacks into cold and heat types may parallel modern medicine's classification of asthma into extrinsic and intrinsic types. Generally speaking, patients with extrinsic asthma often have a cold syndrome, whereas patients with intrinsic asthma typically have a respiratory infection which is frequently manifested as a heat syndrome. The overlap is not complete, however, since these classifications are founded on different theoretical bases.

During remission, the lungs, spleen or kidneys are often in a deficiency state, and the syndrome patterns are classified accordingly. Deficiency of the lungs is characterized by spontaneous sweating and a susceptibility to catching a cold that induces asthmatic attacks. Deficiency of the spleen is characterized by frequent expectoration, lassitude, anorexia, abdominal distension after meals and loose bowel movements. Improper diet usually precipitates asthma attacks. Deficiency of the kidneys is characterized by shortness of breath, a condition which is exacerbated upon exertion, accompanied by aching of the loins and limpness of the legs. Patients with chronic airway obstruction usually have such a syndrome. This syndrome can be further divided into deficiency of kidney-*yin* and deficiency of kidney-*yang*. The former is marked by a dry throat, reddened tongue and thready pulse, the latter by cold extremities, aversion to cold, a pale tongue and a deep, weak pulse.

# TREATMENT

## Herbal medication

It is a general rule of herbal medication that during the asthmatic attack the physician should give precedence to the use of antiasthmatics for symptomatic relief. He should also administer warming drugs in cases of cold type asthma to dispel pathogenic cold and cooling drugs in cases of heat type asthma to remove pathogenic heat. It is also important to administer phlegm eliminating drugs because accumulation of phlegm is considered the basic cause of asthma. Therefore, a traditional prescription for treating an asthmatic episode will consist of at least three parts: antiasthmatics, phlegm-eliminating drugs and cold-dispelling or heat-removing drugs.

After the episode is over, treatment should reinforce the functions of the lungs, spleen and/or kidneys.

The herbal drugs commonly used for treating asthmatic attacks are described below. They usually constitute the ingredients of a compound prescription.

1. Antiasthmatic drugs: *Herba Ephedrae* (ephdra 麻黃 *mahuang*), *Semen Armeniacae Amarum* (bitter apricot kernel 苦杏仁 *kuxingren*), *Fructus Perillae* (perilla seed 紫蘇子 *zisuzi*), *Flos Daturae* (datura flower 洋金花 *yangjinhua*), *Fructus Aristolochiae* (aristolochia fruit 馬兜鈴 *madouling*) and *Cortex Mori* (mulberry bark 桑白皮 *sangbaipi*).

2. Phlegm-eliminating drugs: *Rhizoma Pinelliae Praeparata* (pinellia tuber 半夏 *banxia*), *Herba Asari* (asarum herb 細辛 *xixin*) and *Semen Lepidii* (lepidium seed 亭藶子 *tinglizi*).

3. Cold-dispelling drugs: *Ramulus Cinnamomi* (cinnamom twigs 桂枝 *guizhi*) and *Rhizoma Zingiberis* (dried ginger 乾薑 *ganjiang*).

4. Heat-removing drugs: *Gypsum Fibrosum* (gypsum 石膏 *shigao*) and *Radix Scutellariae* (scutellaria root 黃芩 *haungqin*).

The herbal drugs indicated for asthma during remission are the same as those used for deficiency syndromes in other disorders. These formulae are described below:

1. Asthmatic episode of the cold type: Dispel cold, eliminate phlegm and relieve asthma. Xiaoqinglong Tang (Minor Decoction of Green Dragon*) is generally used. The composition of this formula and the role of each ingredient will be discussed later.

2. Asthmatic episode of the heat type: Remove heat, eliminate phlegm and relieve asthma. The formula of choice is Dingchuan Tang (Antiasthmatic Decoction), in which *Semen Ginkgo, Herba Ephedrae, Fructus Perillae* and *Semen Armeniaecae Amarus* are antiasthmatics; *Flos Farfarae* and *Rhizoma Pinelliae Praeparata* are added for the

---

* "Green Dragon" is a deity in Chinese mythology (Cf. Neptune among Roman deities). In traditional Chinese medicine, naming a formula after a deity was a way of indicating the formula's extraordinary effect.

elimination of phlegm; and *Radix Scutellariae* and *Cortex Mori* are used for removing heat from the lungs.

3. Asthma during remission: There are three categories of formulae commonly used, i.e., formulae to reinforce the lungs, to invigorate the spleen and to replenish the kidneys.

(1) Yupingfeng San (Jade-screen Powder*) is widely used to replenish vital energy so as to consolidate the body's superficial resistance and to check excessive spontaneous perspiration caused by deficiency of lung-*qi*, which renders one susceptible to cold. Therefore, this formula is indicated for asthmatic patients with lung deficiency syndrome. It is composed of *Radix Astragali*, *Rhizoma Atractylodis Macrocephalae* and *Radix Ledebouriellae*. *Radix Atragali* is the principal ingredient. *Rhizoma Atractylodis Macrocephalae* strengthens the effect of *Radix Astragali* in replenishing vital energy, and *Radix Ledebouriellae* helps protect the body from attack by cold and draughts.

Liujunzi Wan (Pills of Six Noble Ingredients) is representative of formulae that invigorate the function of the spleen. It is indicated for asthmatic patients with spleen deficiency syndrome. It contains *Radix Codonopsis Pilosulae*, Poria, *Rhizoma Atractyloids Macrocephalae*, *Radix Glycyrrhizae Praeparata*, *Pericarpium Reticulatae* and *Rhizoma Pinelliae Praeparata*. The first four ingredients invigorate the function of the spleen, the latter two eliminate phlegm.

Liuwei Dihuang Wan (Pills of Six Drugs with Rehmannia) replenish kidney-*yin*; Shenqi Wan (Pills for Restoring Energy of the Kidney) invigorates kidney-*yang*. Both are commonly used in asthmatic patients with kidney deficiency and are indicated for deficiency of kidney-*yin* (vital essence) and insufficiency of kidney-*yang* (vital function), respectively.

Acupuncture treatment

Chief points: Feishu (BL 13), Hegu (LI 4), Dingchuan (from T1 to T6, 0.5 *cun* lateral to each vertebra, 12 points in total) and Kongzui (LU 6).

Points used in combination: Tiantu (CV 22), Fenglong (ST 40), Neiguan (PC 6) and Tanzhong (CV 17).

Manipulation: Uniform reinforcing-reducing method of acupuncture. Moxibustion may be applied to Feishu (BL 13) and Fengmen (BL 12) at the same time for 15-20 minutes.

## MODERN RESEARCH

Modern medical science only partially understands the pathogenesis of asthma. Initial exposure to an allergen (antigen) in a subject with the appropriate genetic constitution causes the production of a highly reactive "reaginic" antibody that attaches itself to the cells in the bronchi. Evidence has accumulated that reaginic antibodies belong to the IgE class. When the appropriate antigen combines with the cell-fixed IgE, chemical mediators including histamine, slow-reacting substance of anaphylaxis (SRS-A), platelet activating factor, serotonin, bradykinin and prostaglandins are released by mast cells and cause increase secretions, mucosal edema and bronchial smooth muscle

---

* A screen is an upright framework used as protection from draughts. Jade implies great value and solidness. This formula is so named for its efficacy in consolidating the superficial resistance of the body to protect against attack by cold and draughts.

spasms. In addition, the parasympathetic mediator — acetylcholine — is involved in initiating bronchospasms, in which vagally mediated reflex plays an important role.

Thus, the immunochemical pathogenesis of asthma involves the following factors: Production of IgE, release of mediators and biological activity of the released mediators.

In recent years, researchers have studied traditional herbal asthma medications. They have found that some herbal drugs effectively control production of IgE and release of mediators. For example, *Radix Glycyrrhizae* (liquorice) inhibits the reproduction of IgE in sensitization of animals; *Radix Scutellariae* (scutellaria root) inhibits the enzyme activity that is necessary for degranulation of mast cells and release of histamine and SRS-A. Some herbal drugs also have antagonistic actions against the biological activity of the mediators implicated in asthma. *Herba Ephedrae* (ephedra) is effective against histamine induced bronchospasms, and *Herba Asari* (asarum herb) against acetylcholine induced bronchospasms.

It is interesting to compare traditional knowledge and modern scientific understanding of the action of Xiaoqinglong Tang (Minor Decoction of Green Dragon) in treating asthma (see Table IX-I). Administering compound prescriptions are evidently better than administering a single ingredient since the compounds deliver multiple actions.

Because ephedrine is effective in treating allergic reactioos and asthma, it is natural to attribute the antiasthmatic effect of Xiaoqinglong Tang (Minor Decoction of Green Dragon) to Herba Ephedrae, which contains ephedrine. Indeed, *Herba Ephedrae* is one of the principal ingredients in this formula. However, some other ingredients are also affective in relieving asthma. Experiments using guinea pigs with asthma induced by inhalation of a mixture of acetylcholine chloride and histamine phosphate showed that Minor Decoction of Green Dragon without *Herba Ephedrae* and *Rhizoma Pinelliae Praeparata* had therapeutic effects similar to the Decoction with all the ingredients.

**Table IX-I. Comparison between the Traditional and Modern Understandings of the Actions of Xiaoqinglong Tang (Minor Decoction of Green Dragon)**

| Ingredients | Traditional | Modern |
|---|---|---|
| *Herba Ephedrae* (ephedra) | Relieves asthma and causes diaphoresis | Relieves bronchosopasms induced by Ach |
| *Ramulus Cinnamomi* (cinnamon twigs) | Dispels cold by increasing perspiratioon | Inhibits degranulation of mast cells and release of mediators |
| *Herba Asari* (asarum herb) | Dispels cold | Relieves bronchospasms induced by H |
| *Rhizoma Zingiberis* (dried ginger) | Dispels cold | |
| *Rhizoma Pinelliae* (pinellia tuber) | Eliminates phlegm | |
| *Fructus Schisandrae* (schisandra fruit) | Relieves asthma | Relieves bronchospasms induced by Ach |
| *Radix Paeoniae Alba* (white peony root) | Checks excessive sweating | Relieves bronchospasms induced by Ach |
| *Radix Glycyrrhizae* (liquorice) | Modulates the actions of other ingredients | Inhibits the production of IgE and degranulation of mast cells |

Ach = Acetylcholine; H = Histamine; IgE = Immumoglobulin E

The herbal formulae indicated for asthmatic patients during remission have no immediate antiasthmatic effect, but they are effective in preventing subsequent asthmatic episodes. Long-term administration of this kind of medicine can improve a patient's constitution, enhance his or her adaptibility to changes in the weather and render one less susceptible to colds. These results suggest that these medicines may effect human immunity.

The effects of Yupingfeng San (Jade-screen Powder) on immunity has already been demonstrated. It acts as a bidirectional immune modulator, both enhancing an insufficient immune reaction and palliating an exaggerated one. *Radix Astragali* (astragalus root), the principal ingredient in this formula, is responsible for this immunological activity.

Liuwei Dihuang Wan (Pills of Six Drugs with Rehmannia) and the first four ingredients of Liujunzi Wan (Pills of Six Noble Ingredients), which is also called Sijunzi Wan (Pills of Four Noble Ingredients), have also been studied from an immunological point of view. Convincing data have been obtained to indicate the modulatory effect of these formulae on human immunity. However, none of these three formulae have been studied in regard to their immunological effect on asthmatic patients.

Researchers have studied some of the kidney tonics (including kidney-tonifying formulae) from an endocrinological standpoint. They found that these formulae stimulated the pituitary-adrenocortical function. Furthermore, researchers found diminished adrenocortical function in asthmatics, especially in those with kidney-*yang* deficiency. Administering appropriate herbal medicines restored the normal adrenocortical function and resulted in clinical improvement. These findings may give some clue as to the therapeutic mechanism of kidney tonics used in asthmatics during remission for prevention of subsequent attacks.

Based on the data obtained through modern research on herbal drugs used in treating asthma and other allergic diseases, doctors developed a new formula in the early 1980s which consists of *Radix Scutellariae* (scutellaria root 黄芩 *huangqin*), *Radix Glycyrrhizae* (liquorice 甘草 *gancao*), *Cortex Moutan* (moutan bark 牡丹皮 *mudanpi*) and *Ramulus Cinnamomi* (cinnamon twig 桂枝 *guizhi*). It is available in decoction or extract form for oral administration. First called "Antiallergic Mixture" and later renamed Xiaochuanning (Antiasthmatic Mixture), it is a slow-acting agent, suitable for long-term control of repeated attacks rather than immediate relief from a severe acute attack. Severe acute attacks may require transient additional use of bronchodilators (e.g., injection of aminophylline). The new formula has shown great promise. In a study of 158 asthmatic cases with frequent attacks treated with Xiaochuanning for half a month, the attacks were totally or basically controlled in 53.2 precent of the cases and the total effective rate was 77.2 percent. In the control group treated with a placebo, total or basic control of the attacks occurred in only 13.3 percent of the cases. Better results were obtained in the extrinsic type of asthma (cold type of asthma according to traditional diagnosis), but considerable effect was also shown in the intrinsic or heat type, as well as in asthmatic bronchitis. Furthermore, 50 percent of the patients who received Xiaochuanning in the appropriate season before the episodes avoided any asthmatic attacks. Clinical observations has thus far revealed no side effects.

Pharmacological studies have shown that the main mechanism of Xiaochuanning in treating asthma is suppression of SRS-A release and antagonism against its activity. In addition, *Radix Scutellariae* acts against histamine and acetylcholine, and *Cortex Mou-*

*tan* against histamine. Research has further shown that Xiaochuanning can suppress not only Type I allergic reactions (as seen in allergic asthma) but also Type III (serum sickness-like) and Type IV (delayed) allergic reactions. This agent seems to have a specific effect on allergic reactions but does not suppress normal immunity, either cellular or humoral.

Success in preventing asthmatic attacks with kidney tonics is probably more significant than the discovery of antiallergic agents in herbal medicine. Use of kidney tonics in treating asthma is a unique feature of traditional Chinese medicine. Clinical observations have repeatedly confirmed the effect of this peculiar method of medication. For instance, Shen, et al., of Shanghai Medical University reported that satisfactory results with control or marked amelioration of the attacks were obtained in 57.5 percent of the 45 asthmatics treated with kidney tonics for about six months each year for three consecutive years. However, in the control group of 19 asthmatics, who received no treatment other than symptomatic relief using aminophylline and ephedrine, satisfactory results were seen in only 10.6 percent of the cases. Repetitive observations on other patients in the same way during the following three consecutive years showed similar results.

In the light of these observations, physicians developed a new formula for a kidney tonic to invigorate the vital function of the kidneys. It is called Wenyang Pian (Kidney Tonic Tablet for *Yang* Deficiency) and is composed of *Radix Aconiti Lateralis Praeparata* (prepared aconite    附子 *fuzi*), *Radix Rehmanniae* (rehmannia root    地黄 *dihuang*), *Rhizoma Dioscoreae* (Chinese yam    山藥 *shanyao*), *Herba Epimedii* (epidemium 淫羊藿 *yinyangsuo*), *Fructus Psoraleae* (psoralea fruit    補骨脂 *buguzhi*) and *Semen Cuscutae* (dodder seed    菟絲子 *tusizi*). Hu,et al., of Shanghai Medical University reported the preventive effect of Wenyang Pian observed in a group of 60 asthmatic patients with a history of seasonal attacks starting from October every year. Doctors there administered Wenyang Pian in these cases from August to October for at least one-and-a-half months. They gave Xiaoqinglong Tang to another group of 36 asthmatics for the same period of time as the control group. Seventy-five percent of the former group achieved satisfactory results but only 19.5 percent of the latter group did. Serum IgE was assayed in this study, for asthmatic patients with seasonal episodes usually have parallel variations in serum IgE concentration. In July the average serum IgE concentration was similar in the two groups, whereas in October the control group showed a marked elevation of serum IgE concentration but the Wenyang Pian group showed no change. The authors obtained similar results in repeat observations and proposed that suppression of the seasonal elevation of serum IgE might be responsible for the effect of Wenyang Pian in controlling subsequent attacks.

The therapeutic mechanisms of Wenyang Pian and other kidney tonics require further investigation. However, there has been enough evidence to suggest that they are not immumnosuppressive agents, nor do they act like corticosteroids so far as their influence on immunity is concerned. They do not suppress normal immune reactions; on the contrary, they promote normal immune reactions when these reactions are at a lowered level. Therefore, successful use of kidney tonics in treating asthma has opened up a new approach to the effective management of asthmatic patients.

# CHAPTER X   GASTRITIS

Gastritis, or inflammation of the stomach mucosa, may be diffuse, involving all parts of the stomach, or localized to a specific area.

Gastritis is classified as acute or chronic primarily on the basis of histologic and/or endoscopic findings and the clinical course of the disease. Acute gastritis is believed to be a self-limited disease, whereas chronic gastritis by definition persists for a long period.

Acute gastritis is characterized by epigastric pain, nausea and vomiting, and in severe cases accompanied by hematemesis and/or melena.

Chronic gastritis includes three categories divided on the basis of mucosal histologic changes: superficial gastritis, chronic atrophic gastritis and gastric atrophy (a severe form of atrophic gastritis). Chronic gastritis shares the same symptoms as acute gastritis. However, because epigastric pain is the main symptom of chronic gastritis, traditional treatment has focused on the principles for differentiating the syndromes of epigastric pain.

## ETIOLOGY AND PATHOGENESIS

The following pathogenic factors cause epigastric pain:

**1. Impairment of the spleen and stomach by improper diet**

Irregular food intake, overeating or hunger, as well as ingestion of unclean, decayed and poisonous food, can all impair the *qi* of both the spleen and stomach. Improper diet includes overindulgence in raw or cold food that causes pathogenic cold to accumulate and both *qi* and blood to stagnate in the stomach, and consumption of too much greasy food or alcoholic drink that produces damp-heat in the spleen and stomach. These pathogenic factors disturb stomach *qi*, which fails to descend, resulting in its stagnation, and hence epigastric pain. The etiology and pathogenesis of acute gastritis usually falls under this category.

**2. Affection of the stomach by hyperactive liver *qi***

Anxiety, anger and mental depression injure the liver, causing liver *qi* to stagnate, which affects the normal function of the stomach and the descending of stomach *qi*, resulting in stomachache. This morbid state is usually called "incoordination between the liver and the stomach." If the liver *qi* remains depressed for a long time, it may turn to heat, which will consume stomach *yin*, producing the syndrome of stomach *yin* deficiency.

**3. Deficiency cold of the spleen and stomach**

Pathogenic factors, such as overstrain and stress, prolonged illness and improper medical treatment, as well as a congenital defect in the *yang* of both the spleen and stomach cause this morbid state. These pathogenic factors damage the transporting and transforming functions of the spleen and the descending function of the stomach, resulting in accumulation of pathogenic damp in the spleen and stomach, and hence epigastric pain.

Generally speaking, the etiology and pathogenesis of chronic gastritis usually falls under the latter two categories.

# DIFFERENTIAL DIAGNOSIS OF SYNDROMES

### 1. Impairment of the spleen and stomach by improper diet

Primary manifestations: Sudden onset of severe epigastric pain aggravated by pressure and alleviated by warmth, belching with fetid odour or vomiting of undigested food, poor appetite, thick, sticky tongue coating and taut and tight or rolling pulse. It should be noted that long-standing cases of pathogenic cold may turn to heat. In these cases, the symptoms of damp heat may appear, such as dry mouth with no desire for drink and reddened tongue with yellow, greasy coating.

### 2. Attack of the stomach by hyperactive liver *qi*

Primary manifestations: Pain and distension in the epigastric region radiating to the bilateral hypochondriac regions, distress in the chest and belching aggravated by anxiety and mental depression, irritability, thin, white tongue coating and taut pulse. Liver *qi* stagnated for a long term may turn to heat, which causes severe pain accompanied by acid regurgitation, dry mouth with bitter taste, reddened tongue with yellow, greasy coating and taut, rapid pulse. Pathogenic heat may also consume *yin* and lead to *yin* deficiency of the spleen and stomach.

### 3. Deficiency cold of the spleen and stomach

Primary manifestations: Continuous dull pain in the upper abdomen, preference for pressure and warmth, loss of appetite, vomiting of clear fluid, lassitude, cool limbs, pale and flabby tongue with teeth prints along its borders, thin, white tongue coating and weak, thready pulse.

### 4. Blood stasis in the collaterals

Primary manifestations: Localized stabbing pain or tenderness aggravated by pressure, vomiting of blood, melena, dark-purplish tongue or with purple dots on it and hesitant pulse.

### 5. *Yin* deficiency of the spleen and stomach

Primary manifestations: Dull stomachache with burning feeling, dry throat and thirst with preference for cold beverages, constipation, reddened tongue with thin and yellow coating or absence of coating and small and rapid pulse or taut and small pulse.

# TREATMENT

### 1. Impairment of the spleen and stomach by improper diet

Principle of treatment: Expel the pathogenic cold, promote digestion and relieve food retention.

1) Formula of choice: Liang Fu Wan (Galangal and Cyperus Pill) is indicated

in accummulation of cold in the stomach; in this formula, *Rhizoma Galangae* (galangal rhizome) expels the pathogenic cold from the stomach; *Rhizoma Cyperi* (cyperus tuber) promotes the descending of the stomach *qi*; they are used in combination to relieve epigastric pain; the formula is usually made into a decoction for treating acute stomachache; if pathogenic cold is marked, *Rhizoma Zingiberis* (dried ginger) and *Fructus Evodiae* (evodia fruit) may be added to strengthen the effect of warming the stomach; if the stagnation of *qi* is predominant, *Pericarpium Citri Reticulatae* (tangerine peel) and *Radix Aucklandiae* (aucklandia root) may be used to activate the flow of *qi*; if the epigastric pain is accompanied by chills and fever, *Rhizoma Zingiberis Recens* (fresh ginger) and *Herba Agastachi* (agastache) are added to expel the wind and cold.

2) Baohe Wan (Lenitive Pill) is used to treat stomachache due to retention of food; it promotes digestion, pacifies the stomach and relieves pain; the usual dosage is 2 pills 3 times a day, but it may also be made into decoction for acute cases.

3) Decoction for Purging Stomach Fire is adopted if there is damp-heat in the spleen and stomach.

**2. Attack of the stomach by hyperactive liver *qi***

Principle of treatment: Disperse the depressed liver *qi* and regulate stomach *qi*.

Formula of choice: Chaihu Shugan San (Bupleurum Powder for Relieving Liver *Qi*), in which *Radix Paeoniae, Rhizoma Ligustici Chuanxiong, Radix Bupleuri, Fructus Auranti* and *Rhizoma Cyperi* regulate liver *qi* and *Pericarpium Citri Reticulatae* and *Radix Glycyrrhizae Praeparata* regulate stomach *qi*; if the depressed liver *qi* turns into heat, *Fructus Gardeniae* and *Cortex Moutan Radicis* should be added (Note: Because drugs that regulate liver *qi* are pungent in flavor and warm in property, which may consume *yin* of the liver and stomach, these drugs should not be used in overdosage and for too long; if there are heat signs, it is better to use these drugs together with drugs that nourish liver blood and stomach *yin*).

**3. Deficiency cold of the spleen and stomach**

Principle of treatment: Tonify the spleen and stomach and expel the cold.

Formula of choice: Huangqi Jianzhong Tang (Decoction of Astragalus for Tonifying Middle-*Jiao*), which warms and tonifies *qi* of the spleen and stomach and relieves pain; if pain is severe, *Rhizoma Alpiniae Officinarum, Rhizoma Zingiberis* and *Rhizoma Cyperi* may be added; after the pain is basically relieved, Xiangsha Liujunzi Tang (Decoction of Aucklandia and Amomum with Six Noble Ingredients) can be adopted to adjust and restore the function of the spleen and stomach.

**4. Blood stasis in the collaterals**

Principle of treatment: Promote blood circulation and eliminate blood stasis; it is necessary to determine whether the blood stasis is caused by *qi* stagnation or *qi* deficiency; in the former type, the principle of treatment is to regulate the flow of *qi* and to remove the blood in order to relieve pain; the latter type should be treated with drugs that replenish *qi* and promote blood circulation.

Formula of choice:

1) Sini San (Powder for Treating Cold Limbs) or Shixiao San (Wonderful Powder

for Relieving Blood Stagnation) in cases of blood stasis caused by *qi* stagnation; in these formulae *Radix Bupleuri* and *Fructus Aurantii Immaturus* adjust liver *qi*, and *Radix Paeoniae Alba*, *Pollen Typhae* and *Faeces Trogopterorum* promote blood circulation and remove blood stasis.

2) Liang Fu Wan (Galangal and Cyperus Pill) in addition to Decoction of Invigorating *Yang* for Recuperation in cases of blood stasis caused by *qi* deficiency; in this formula *Radix Astragali* is the principal ingredient for invigorating *qi*, *Rhizoma Galangae* and *Rhizoma Cyperus* warm the stomach and regulate *qi* and the other ingredients remove blood stasis.

**5. *Yin* deficiency of the spleen and stomach**

Principle of treatment: Nourish *yin* and regulate the stomach.

Formula of choice: Yiguan Jian (Ever-effective Decoction for Nourishing the Liver and Kidneys) and Nourishing the Stomach Decoction; in these formulae *Fructus Meliae Toosendan* disperses the stagnated liver *qi*, the other ingredients nourish *yin*; if constipation occurs, add *Semen Trichosanthis*; if dry mouth with bitter taste occurs, add a small dose of *Rhizoma Coptidis* to clear away heat from the stomach; if pain is severe, add *Radix Paeoniae Alba* and *Radix Glycyrrhizae* to relieve spasms and stop pain.

Acupunctrue treatment

Principal acupoints: Zhongwan (CV 12), Neiguan (PC 6) and Zusanli (ST 36); Zusanli (ST 36) is the He (sea) point of the Stomach Meridian, and Zhongwan (CV12) is the Front-Mu point; these two points used together pacify the stomach and activate the descent of *qi*; Neiguan (PC 6) is one of the pair-points of the Eight Confluent points and relieves the fullness of the stomach.

Supplementary points:

1. For accumulation of cold and retention of food in the stomach, add Shangwan (CV 13) and Pishu (BL 20) to eliminate cold and undigested food.

2. If the stomach is attacked by hyperactive liver *qi*, add Qimen (LR 14) and Taichong (LR 3) to remove stagnated liver *qi*, regulate its flow and relieve pain.

3. For deficiency cold of the spleen and stomach, apply acupuncture and moxibustion to Qihai (CV 6), Pishu (BL 20), Gongsun (SP 4) and Zhangmen (LR 13) to warm the spleen and stomach, eliminate cold, regulate the flow of *qi* and relieve pain.

4. For blood stasis in the collaterals, add Geshu (BL 17), Ganshu (BL 18) and Pishu (BL 20) to regulate the flow of *qi* and promote blood circulation.

5. For *yin* deficiency of the spleen and stomach, add Pishu (BL 20), Weishu (BL 21), Sanyinjiao (SP 6) and Taixi (KI 3) to nourish *yin* and clear away heat from the stomach.

# MODERN RESEARCH

As acute gastritis is a self-limited disease, it is difficult to evaluate traditional methods of treating it. However, physicians have conducted a great deal of research on the treatment of chronic gastritis, since modern medicine has no specific therapy to treat it.

Although opinions differ regarding the classification of syndromes in chronic gastritis, most authors consider these the common syndromes: attack of the stomach by hyperactive liver *qi* (also called incoordination between the liver and stomach), deficiency cold of the spleen and stomach, *yin* deficiency of the stomach and blood stasis in the collaterals. Some authors believe that patients with superficial or early chronic gastritis experience incoordination between the liver and the stomach, whereas patients with atrophic or advanced chronic gastritis experience deficiency syndromes.

Because traditional Chinese medicine considers the tongue "the mirror of the stomach," many researchers have focused on the relationship between gastroscopic findings and inspection of the tongue.

Zhan Jianlie, et al., (Longhua Hospital, Shanghai College of Traditional Chinese Medicine) observed the gastroscopic findings in two thousand cases of chronic digestive disease. The authors found superficial atrophic gastritis in 470 cases, atrophic gastritis in 367 cases, gastric ulcer in 174 cases, duodenal ulcer in 211 cases and gastric cancer in 94 cases. In order to investigate the relationship between the gastroscopic findings and the syndrome differentiations, the authors classified the patients into these four syndrome types and their respective gastroscopic findings:

1. Stomach cold in 547 cases (27.4 percent): Gastric mucosa was pale or pink and covered by thin mucus; capillaries were congested and greyish blue.

2. Stomach heat in 597 cases (29.8 percent): Gastric mucosa was deep red with disseminated congestion; congested, purplish capillaries looked like a network; mucosal surface was dry, fragile, coarse and hypertrophic.

3. Attack of the stomach collateral by stagnated *qi* in 484 cases (24.2 percent): Gastric mucosa was dark red with arborizing capillaries, granular or nodular hyperplasia and petechial hemorrhages.

4. Impairment of the stomach collateral by pathogenic heat in 372 cases (18.6 percent): Gastric mucosa was fragile and dark red with disseminated congestion, petechial hemorrhage and erosions, granular hyperplasia and covered with yellow, thick and dirty mucus.

Basing their work on gastroscopic findings, some Chinese physicians are making traditional diagnoses of syndromes in chronic gastritis and selecting appropriate formulae to treat them. For example, Zheng Jingren, et al., (Shanghai First People's Hospital) recommonds *Radix Paeoniae Rubra* and *Fructus Forsythiae* to clear away heat in cases of mucosal erosion or hemorrhage; *Flos Inulae* and *Haematitum* to promote the descending of stomach *qi* when there is reflux of bile; *Herba Oldenlandiae Diffusae* to clear away heat and dissipate masses in cases of intestinal metaplasia; *Radix Salviae Miltiorrhiae*, *Radix Paeoniae Rubra* and *Radix Angelicae Sinensis* to promote blood circulation and remove blood stasis if the gastric mucosa is pale and the number of mucous glands has decreased. They also reported on the effects of a formula composed of *Caulis Perillae*, *Rhizoma Cyperi*, *Radix Paeoniae Alba*, *Radix Glycyrrhizae* and *Rhizoma Atractylodis Macrocephalae* in treating 122 patients with chronic gastritis. After three months' treatment, the total effective rate was 87.7 percent. In 32 cases of intestinal metaplasia, the histological changes improved in all cases, and intestinal metaplasia disappeared in 10 cases after treatment.

Chu Hang, et al., (First Affiliated Hospital, China Medical University, Shenyang) reported on 106 cases of chronic gastritis treated by replenishing *qi* and removing blood stasis. Another 30 cases were chosen randomly as a control group and were treated with a placebo (dried yeast). The effective rate in the experimental group was 88.3 percent and 6.7 percent in the control group. Doctors repeated the gastroscopy on 32 cases in the experimental group after treatment and found that 15 cases (46.9 percent) showed gastroscopic improvement, and 17 cases (53.1 percent) showed histological improvement.

Zhu Yunhua, et al., (Jiangsu Provincial Traditional Chinese Medicine Hospital) observed the relationship between the syndromes of traditional Chinese medicine and infection caused by campylobacter pyloridis (CP) in 100 patients with chronic gastritis. The patients were divided into two groups: Group I included 57 cases of deficiency of the middle-*jiao* and stagnation of *qi*; Group II included 36 cases of disharmony of the liver and the stomach and seven cases of deficiency of stomach *yin*. The pathohistologic investigation and urease test showed that the CP infection rate was 92.9 percent in Group I, but 58.1 percent in Group II. Pharmacological study revealed that *Rhizoma Coptidis, Radix et Rhizoma Rhei, Fructus Mume, Radix Salviae Miltiorrhizae* and *Radix Notoginseng* effectively inhibited campylobacter pylordis.

Feng Yangzheng, et al., (Institute of Industrial Health, the National Mechanical Industry Commission) reported on 103 cases of chronic atrophic gastritis treated with Daoyin-Tuna Qigong therapy (a special kind of Qigong exercise combined with massage). Patients performed the exercise four times a day, one hour each time, for 79 days. After the treatment, symptomatic improvement was seen in 97.1 percent of the cases, and the effective rates on gastroscopy and pathohistology were 64.5 percent and 87.1 percent, respectively.

Gao Shouzheng, et al., (Beijing Jishuitan Hospital) reported on 408 patients with chronic superficial gastritis diagnosed by fibrogastroscopy and histology that were divided into two groups randomly: 325 patients in Group A received Weining Granules (consisting of *Radix Codonopsis Pilosulae*, Poria, *Rhizoma Atractylodis Macrocephalae, Radix Aucklandiae, Fructus Meliae Toosendan, Fructus Mume,* etc.), 20 g three times a day for three months; 83 patients in Group B received a placebo, by single blind trial. In Group A symptomatic, gastroscopic and histologic effective rates were 90.5 percent, 81.9 percent and 72.8 percent, respectively, while in Group B they were 50.6 percent, 46.3 percent and 16.7 percent, respectively. Other experiments have shown that Weining Granules protect the gastric mucous membrane in rats and guinea pigs. In animals with drug-induced gastritis and gastric ulcer, the effect of Weining Granules was similar to Cimetidin. Other pharmacological studies have proven that Weining Granules inhibit pepsin secretion. These findings have established Weining Granules as an alternative to H2-receptor inhibitor as a treatment for chronic superficial gastritis.

Zhou Zuhua (Geriatric Research Institute of Hunan Province, Changsha) reported on 150 cases of chronic superficial gastritis diagnosed on the basis of gastroscopic and pathohistological findings. Zhou randomly divided the patients into two groups (60 male and 15 female in each group). Patients in Group I received Wei Yan Kang (a preparation for "recovery from gastritis," consisting of *Radix Glycyrrhizae, Radix Paeoniae, Ramulus Cinnamomi, Rhizoma Alpiniae Officinarum, Rhizoma Coptidis* and *Radix Bupleuri*). Those in Group II received Cimetidin. Wei Yan Kang dosage was 4 g twice a day and that of Cimetidin 1 g daily during the first month and 0.4 g every night during the second and third months. The effective rates of gastroscopic observation, gastric biopsy and symptomatic improvement for Group I were 73.3 percent, 68.4 percent and 86.0 percent, respectively, and for Group II 68.0 percent, 61.1 percent and 93.3 percent, respectively. Zhou followed 41 cases in Group I and 40 cases in Group II over two years and found that symptoms recurred in 63.4 percent of the Group I cases and 90.0 percent of the Group II cases. The recurrence rate of severe symptoms was 19.5 percent in Group I and 45.0 percent in Group II. The results indicate that in the long-term Wei Yan Kang may be even more effective than Cimetidin in treating chronic superficial gastritis.

# CHAPTER XI    PEPTIC ULCER

Peptic ulcers occur in the stomach, pylorus and duodenal bulb. They can also develop in the esophagus and the postbulbar doudenum.

The digestive action of hydrochloric acid and pepsin on the mucosa causes ulcers in the upper gastrointestinal tract. Thus, these became known as "peptic ulcers." The clinical manifestations of peptic ulcer are epigastric pain with a feeling of fullness, nausea, vomiting and anorexia. The clinical diagnosis of peptic ulcer is based primarily on the location and character of pain. Ulcer pain is classically described as located in the epigastrium, burning or gnawing in character, and relieved by taking food or antacids. The pain occurs in episodes lasting from days to weeks, interspersed with long symptom-free periods. But the definite diagnosis of peptic ulcer depends on visualizing the ulcer crater using radigoraphy or the ulcer lesion using endoscopy.

In traditional Chinese medicine, peptic ulcer is closely associated with "epigastric pain" in syndrome diagnosis and treatment.

## ETIOLOGY AND PATHOGENESIS

The etiology and pathogenesis of epigastric pain have been described in Chapter X, which deals with gastritis. The following discussion focuses on the clinical features of peptic ulcer.

In most cases of peptic ulcer the basic pathologic condition is deficiency cold of the spleen and stomach. Pain often occurs after eating cold food or when the stomach is empty, and is alleviated by warm food or by pressure. In addition, pain often recurs during cool or cold seasons. Thus, the pathogenesis of peptic ulcer is deficiency of spleen *yang* leading to the production of endogenic cold, which hinders the spleen's transmission and transformation of food and the descending of stomach *qi*. In some cases, stagnated liver *qi* may complicate the deficiency-cold of the spleen and stomach syndrome. This adversely affects the stomach and may turn into heat or lead to blood stasis.

## DIFFERENTIAL DIAGNOSIS OF SYNDROMES

### 1. Deficiency-cold of the spleen and stomach
Primary manifestations: Dull epigastric pain alleviated by pressure and warmth or relieved after eating, vomiting of watery fluid, lassitude, cool limbs, pale and flabby tongue with thin white coating or teeth prints along its borders and weak and fine pulse. This syndrome often recurs during cold seasons.

### 2. Attack of stagnated liver *qi* on the stomach
Primary manifestations: Distending pain in the epigastric region, acid regurgitation and belching, aggravated by anxiety and mental depression, thin, white tongue coating

and taut pulse.

If stagnated liver *qi* lasts for a long time, it may turn into heat, manifested as thirst, reddened tongue with yellow coating and rapid and taut pulse.

Stagnated liver *qi* may also cause blood stasis, which is characterized by localized stabbing pain aggravated by pressure, dark purple tongue or with petechiae, thin, white tongue coating and hesitant pulse.

### 3. Accumulation of phlegm-damp in the middle-*jiao*

Primary manifestations: Epigastric pain occurring after meals, thirst without preference for drink, poor appetite, white and greasy tongue coating and smooth pulse. These symptoms indicate a phlegm-damp syndrome of the cold type. If the tongue becomes red with a yellow and greasy coating and the patient experiences thirst, concentrated urine and constipation, the phlegm-damp syndrome has turned into damp-heat.

## TREATMENT

### 1. Deficiency-cold of the spleen and stomach

Principle of treatment: Strengthen the middle-*jiao* and warm the stomach.

Formula of choice: Huangqi Jianzhong Tang (Astragalus Decoction for Tonifying the Middle-*jiao*), a famous prescription for strengthening and warming the spleen and stomach to relieve epigastric pain; in this formula *Radix Astragali* strengthens the *qi* of the middle-*jiao*, *Ramulus Cinnamomi* warms the middle-*jiao* and eliminates pathogenic cold and *Radix Paeoniae Alba* together with *Radix Glycyrrhizae Praeparata* relieve spasms and pain; the original formula includes *Rhizoma Zingiberis Recens* which may be replaced by *Rhizoma Zingiberis Praeparata*; malt sugar can also be added to warm and invigorate the middle-*jiao*, but if acid regurgitation is present, malt sugar should be given in small dosages or totally subtracted; *Os Sepiellae Seu Sepiae* or *Rhizoma Pinelliae Praeparata* and *Pericarpium Citri Reticulatae* can be added to regulate the stomach function and keep the stomach *qi* going downwards.

### 2. Attack of stagnated liver *qi* on the stomach

Principle of treatment: Disperse stagnated liver *qi* and harmonize the stomach.

Formula of choice: Chaihu Shugan San (Bupleurum Powder for Soothing the Liver); if the syndrome is complicated by blood stasis, *Rhizoma Corydalis*, *Radix Salviae Miltiorrhizae* and *Faeces Trogopterorum* may be added to promote blood circulation and eliminate blood stasis.

### 3. Accumulation of phlegm-damp in the middle-*jiao*

Principle of treatment: Strengthen the spleen and eliminate phlegm-damp.

Formula of choice: Erchen Decoction (Decotion of Two Old Drugs) and Liang Fu Wan (Galangal and Cyperus Pill); Poria and *Radix Glycyrrhizae Praeparata* strengthen the spleen and dispel damp; *Rhizoma Pinelliae Praeparata* is used with Poria and *Radix Glycyrrhizae* to strengthen the effect of dispelling phlegm-damp; *Pericarpium Citri Reticulatae*, *Rhizoma Cyperi* and *Rhizoma Alpiniae* regulate *qi* and relieve pain; if the phlegm-damp has turned into phlegm-heat, it should be treated with Banxia Xiexin Tang (Pinellia Decoction for Purging Stomach Fire); in this formula, *Rhizoma Coptidis* and *Radix Scutellariae* dispel internal heat, *Rhizoma Zingiberis* and *Rhizoma Pinelliae* dispel phlegm and *Radix Ginseng, Radix Glycyrrhizae Praeparata* and *Fructus Ziziphi Jujubae* strengthen the spleen and harmonize the stomach

The therapeutic principles and formulae as well as the acupuncture points described in Chapter X on gastritis are also recommended for treating peptic ulcers based on differentiation of syndromes.

## MODERN RESEARCH

Pang Ninghai, et al., (First Affiliated Hospital, Beijing Medicial University) have observed the nature of cold and heat syndromes in 62 patients with peptic ulcer. They classified these patients into three categories: heat syndrome (23 cases), cold syndrome (16 cases) and unapparent heat or cold syndrome (23 cases). The authors conducted tests to determine urine catecholamines (CAs) in these patients and 26 healthy persons. CAs were above normal in heat syndrome cases, below normal in cold syndrome cases and practically normal in unapparent heat or cold syndrome cases. These findings suggest hyperfunctioning of the sympathetic-adrenomedullary system in heat syndromes and hypofunctioning of the sympathetic system in cold syndromes. After receiving herbal medication, patients showed clinical improvement and their CAs in heat and cold syndromes returned to normal. This indicates that dysfunction of the sympathetic-adrenal system is one of the fundamental changes upon which the differentiation of cold and heat syndromes is founded. The regulation or correction of this disordered functional state is one of the main principles in traditional Chinese medicine.

Wang Jiuchun, et al., (General Hospital of the Jinan Command of the People's Liberation Army) reported on 180 hospitalized patients with peptic ulcer who were randomly divided into three groups. Group A contained 60 cases. They received herbal medicine according to differentiation of syndromes. Group B had 60 cases, who received antacids and antispasmodics, such as aluminum hydroxide and probenzin, but no H2 receptor antagonist. Group C's 60 cases received a combination of both traditional Chinese and Western medicine. The cure rates in Groups A, B and C were 55 percent, 41.6 percent and 68.9 percent, respectively. In this instance, combined treatment was most efficacious.

Pu Changsheng, et al., (The Second Affiliated Hospital of Lanzhou Medical College) observed the effects of Peptic Ulcer Table (PUT) on 125 patients with peptic ulcer. This tablet consists of *Kronopolites Svenhedini Verhoeff* (containing 45.18 percent calcium carbonate), *Radix Notoginseng, Radix Saussureae Lappae, Radix Glycyrrhizae, Radix Salviae Miltiorrhizae, Radix Peoniae Alba, Rhizoma Atractylodis Macrocephalae, Rhizoma Corydalis* and *Rhizoma Cyperi*. Another group of 91 peptic ulcer patients served as a control group and received Cimetidin. After four weeks of treatment, patients treated with PUT experienced a cure rate of 64.8 percent. Another 18.4 percent, saw their ulcers reduce in size, for a total effective rate of 83.2 percent. The rates for the group treated with Cimetidin were 69.23 percent, 16.84 percent and 85.71 percent, respectively, indicating that PUT was as effective as Cimetidin without the side effects.

Researchers have also studied the pharmacological actions of drugs and decoctions for replenishing the spleen and invigorating *qi*, such as Ginseng, *Codonopsis Pilosula*,

*Astragalus*, Si Junzi Tang (Decoction of Four Noble Drugs) and Buzhong Yiqi Tang (Decoction for Reinforcing Middle-*jiao* and Replenishing *Qi*). They have found that the main actions of these drugs are regulating and strengthening digestive, immune and neuro-humoral functions as well as energy metabolism. For example, Decoction of Four Noble Drugs promotes the secretion of the pancreas, raises the absorptive rate of xylose, regulates gastric secretions and relieves gastrointestinal spasms. Like atropine, it inhibits the smooth muscle hypertonia caused by acetylcholine and histamine.

# TREATMENT OF COMPLICATIONS

## I. Perforation

Western physicians typically indicate surgery in peptic ulcer patients with perforation, hemorrhage or obstruction. In the past 30 years, however, Chinese physicians have studied the effects of combined traditional Chinese and Western medical treatment of perforated peptic ulcers. This type of treatment is indicated in patients under 60 years old who are in good general condition, have normal blood pressure, pulse and respiration, show no obvious abnormalities of the heart, lungs, liver and kidneys, have had a short course of peptic uler and an absence of shifting dullness in the abdomen and whose body temperature is less than 39 °C. The therapeutic regimen consists of three stages.

First stage: The patient should be in a semi-reclining position; no food intake is allowed. The main treatment includes gastrointestinal decompression, intravenous infusion with antibiotics and electrically stimulated acupuncture. The principal acupoints are Zusanli (ST 36), Zhongwan (CV 16), Tianshu (ST 25) and Liangmen (ST 21). The needles should be retained for 12-24 hours, with electric stimulation every two hours for 30 minutes each time. The patient should be closely observed for 12-24 hours. If the patient's condition improves, the treatment can be continued; otherwise, surgical intervention should be given at once. Experimental studies revealed the multiple effects of acupuncture therapy in this stage: to inhibit the secretion of gastric fluid, acid and pepsin; to promote the restoration of peristalsis and the opening of the pylorus to evacuate the gastric content; and to increase the phagocytic function.

Second stage: Clearing away heat and counteracting toxicity are the main principles of treatment in this stage. Use Da Chaihu Tang (Major Bupleurum Decoction) with modifications for 5-7 days. Its main ingredients are *Radix Bupleuri, Radix Scutellariae, Radix et Rhizoma Rhei, Fructus Aurantii Immaturus, Radix Paeoniae Alba, Cortex Phellodendri, Herba Taraxaci, Radix Aucklandiae, Fructus Meliae Toosendan, Rhizoma Corydalis* and *Radix Glycyrrhizae*. When the patient recovers his appetite, his body temperature will return to normal, his symptoms will basically disappear and he is ready for the third stage of treatment.

Studies have shown that Major Bupleurum Decoction is anti-inflammator and antibiotic, and restores gastrointestinal functions and promotes absorption of abdominal exudate.

Third stage (convalescence): Here treatment is aimed at curing the peptic ulcer. In cases of excess-heat type, the treatment involves clearing heat and purging fire, using

Banxia Xiexin Tang (Pinellia Decoction for Purging Stomach Fire) with modifications. In cases of deficiency-cold type, therapy involves replenishing *qi* and warming middle-*jiao*, using Liu Junzi Tang (Decoction of Six Noble Ingredients) or Lizhong Tang (Decoction for Regulating Middle-*jiao*) with modifications.

In 5,920 cases of ulcerative perforation treated with the combined therapy, the cure rate was 92.4 percent, the mortality rate 0.8 percent. Physicians followed 652 of these cases for five years. Of them, 83.4 percent experienced satisfactory results, while only 11.5 percent needed a gastrectomy.

## II. Hemorrhage

Acute bleeding is another serious complication of peptic ulcers. Here again, traditional Chinese methods combined with Western medical techniques resulted in benefical effects.

Traditional Chinese medicine holds that acute hemorrhage in peptic ulcer is caused by: a) accummulation of heat in the stomach brought on by taking too much heat-propertied food or an attack of pathogenic heat damaging the collaterals of the stomach; b) heat transformed from stagnated liver *qi* attacking the stomach; and c) deficiency of spleen *qi* failing to keep the blood flowing within the vessels.

Differential diagnosis of syndromes and treatment:

1. Bleeding due to accummulation of heat in the stomach

Primary manifestations: Distending pain over the epigastrium and abdomen, hematemesis, thirst with preference for cold drink, scanty urine, constipation, reddened tongue with yellow coating and rapid pulse.

Principle of treatment: Clear away heat from the stomach, remove blood stasis and arrest bleeding.

Formula of choice: Qingwei San (Powder for Clearing Stomach Fire) plus Shihui San (Powder of Ashes of Ten Drugs) with modifications.

2. Bleeding due to the liver heat attacking the stomach

Primary manifestations: Nausea, hematemesis, bitter taste in the mouth, hypochondriac distending pain, irritability, excitability, reddened tongue and taut pulse.

Principle of treatment: Clear away pathogenic heat from the liver and stomach and stop bleeding by cooling the blood.

Formula of choice: Longdan Xiegan Tang (Decoction of Gentian for Purging Liver Fire) plus *Cortex Moutan Radicis*, *Fructus Gardeniae* and *Radix Scutellariae*.

3. Bleeding due to deficiency of spleen and stomach *qi*

Primary manifestations: Pallid complexion, lassitude and weakness, shortness of breath, abdominal distension, nausea, hematemesis, pale tongue and small, deep pulse.

Principle of treatment: Resplenish *qi* to arrest bleeding.

Formula of choice: Guipi Tang (Docoction for Invigorating the Spleen and Nourishing the Heart) with modifications.

In serious cases, the following emergency treatments are recommended in addition to blood transfusions.

1. *Rhizoma Bletillae* Powder (10 g) plus White Drug Powder (2 g): Make into a paste

with 150 ml warm boiled water; 15 ml taken orally every 2 hours on the first day; if the bleeding stops, the dosage may be reduced to 15 ml 4 times a day for 3 days.

2. Rhubarb Powder: 3 g 3 times a day taken orally. Jiao Donghai, et al., (Xianghan Traditional Chinese Medicine Hospital, Shanghai) reported on the use of an alcoholic extract of rhubarb (AER) in treating 182 cases of upper gastrointestinal hemorrhage. AER achieved a total effective rate of 96.1 percent with hemostasis occurring in two-to-eight days. The common causes of bleeding were peptic ulcer, gastritis and neoplasm of the stomach. The mechanisms of AER responsible for hemostasis include contraction of the local blood vessels, reduction in permeability and motility of the small intestine and inhibition of pepsin activity. Elevation of the plasma osmotic pressure may also contribute to hemostasis. Pharmacological studies indicate that rhubarb has two active hemostatic components: d-catechin and gallic acid.

3. Alumen: Wan Kejiang, et al., (Luzhou Medical College, Sichuan) reported on 35 cases of gastric bleeding treated with a 6 percent Alumen Solution which was directly injected to the bleeding sites using gastroscopy. Hemostasis occurred within one minute in 34 cases, and within two minutes in one case. This solution can also be used orally for treating gastric bleeding.

4. *Folium Sennae*: Jin Yacheng, et al., (Hangzhou Third Hospital) reported on the effect of *Folium Sennae* on acute gastroduodenal hemorrhage in 340 cases. A powder of *Folium Sennae* was administered orally at a dose of 1 g 3 times a day. After the treatment, hemostasis occurred in 320 cases (94.1 percent), and the average hemostatic time was $2.68 \pm 0.12$ days, as judged by the absence of occult blood in the feces. A control group of 100 patients received Cimetidin. Their hemostatic rate was 90 percent, and the average hemostatic time was $4.55 \pm 0.16$ days. Experiments showed that coaglation time, thromboplastin time and clot retraction time were remarkably shortened after administering *Folium Sennae*.

# CHAPTER XII CHOLECYSTITIS AND CHOLELITHIASIS

Cholecystitis is an inflammation of the gallbladder, often accompanied by gallstones. Biliary obstruction is usually an initiating factor, while bacterial infection is secondary to it.

Cholecystitis can be acute or chronic. Acute cholecystitis usually begins with a sudden attack of right subcostal pain and tenderness, but two-thirds or more of all patients report having had previous attacks of biliary colic. Fever, anorexia, nausea and vomiting are often present. Chills and high fever suggest suppurative cholecystitis or associated cholangitis. About 20 percent of the patients have mild jaundice. The right subcostal region is tender to palpation with positive Murphy's sign.

Chronic cholecystitis commonly produces a steady pain located in the epigastrium or right upper quadrant of the abdomen, accompanied by nausea and vomiting. The pain subsides gradually to a vague residual ache, or it may remain for a long time. Tenderness, muscular rigidity, palpable masses, fever and leukocytosis are absent. Dyspepsia, flatulence, heartburn and belching may occur.

About thirty-to-fifty percent of patients with gallstones are asymptomatic. The major symptoms are those caused by biliary obstruction and cholecystitis. Ultrasonography is probably the simplest and most reliable method of detecting gallbladder stones in these patients.

Based on their clinical manifestations, cholecystitis and cholelithiasis are linked to the syndromes of "hypochondriac pain" and "jaundice" in traditional Chinese medicine.

## ETIOLOGY AND PATHOGENESIS

### 1. Stagnation of liver *qi*

Emotional stress, worry and anger impede the smooth flow of liver *qi*. As a result, liver *qi* stagnates in the liver and gallbladder, and changes into pathogenic heat. The heat steams the bile, resulting in the formation of gallstones.

### 2. Accumulation of damp-heat

Damp-heat may originate from outside, as a seasonal or epidemic pathogenic factor, or be produced internally, due to impaired spleen and stomach functions caused by improper diet or due to a deficiency state of the spleen which causes its transporting and transforming of water to fail. If, as a result, damp-heat accumulates in the middle-*jiao*, it will steam the liver and gallbladder and cause fever and jaundice.

### 3. Excess of noxious heat

Invasion and accumulation of epidemic noxious heat in the liver and gallbladder impairs *yin*, blood and the pericardium, leading to high fever, jaundice, mental disorder and bleeding.

# DIFFERENTIAL DIAGNOSIS OF SYNDROMES

### 1. Stagnation of liver *qi*

Primary manifestations: Mild and dull pain in the right upper quadrant of the abdomen, bitter taste in the mouth, thirst, jaundice, absence of chills and fever, yellowish tongue coating and normal or taut pulse. This syndrome occurs in patients who have gallstones but no infection or obstruction of the biliary duct, and in some patients with chronic cholecystitis.

### 2. Accumulation of damp-heat

Primary manifestations: Fever, jaundice, nausea, vomiting, pain and tenderness in the right subcostal region, enlarged palpable gallbladder, reddened tongue with yellow, greasy coating and taut and smooth rapid pulse. This syndrome occurs in some cases of acute cholecystitis and cholelithiasis with obvious biliary obstruction and infection.

### 3. Excess of noxious heat

Primary manifestations: (In addition to the manifestations described above in the syndrome of accumulation of damp-heat) Chills, high fever, delirium, impairment of consciousness even coma, reddened tongue with dry, yellow coating and small, rapid pulse. This syndrome occurs in the septic form of acute cholecystitis.

# TREATMENT

### 1. Stagnation of liver *qi*

Principle of treatment: Disperse the depressed liver *qi*, clear away heat and promote the secretion of bile.

Formula of choice: Chaihu Shugan San (Bupleurum Powder for Dispersing the Depressed Liver *Qi*); *Herba Artemisiae Capillaris*, the principal ingredient, combines with *Fructus Gardeniae* to clear away damp-heat and expel jaundice; *Radix et Rhizoma Rhei* purges away stagnated pathogenic heat; Yinchenhao Tang (Oriental Wormwood Decoction) is also used to clear away damp-heat and promote the discharge of bile.

### 2. Accumulation of damp-heat in the liver and gallbladder

Principle of treatment: Clear away heat and eliminate damp from the liver and gallbladder.

Formula of choice: Longdan Xiegan Tang (Decoction of Gentian for Purging Liver-Fire) with modifications; *Radix Gentianae* is strong-bitter in taste and cold in nature to purge the fire in the liver and gallbladder; *Radix Scutellariae* and *Fructus Gardeniae*, bitter in taste and cold in nature, clear away the fire and eliminate damp; *Caulis Clematidis Armandii*, *Semen Plantaginis* and *Rhizoma Alismatis* clear away damp-heat; *Radix Bupleuri* regulates liver *qi*; *Radix Angelicae Sinensis* and *Radix Rehmanniae* protect the liver *yin* and blood from being injured by the pathogenic damp-heat; in cases of serious jaundice, add *Herba Artemisiae Capillaris* and *Herba Lysimachiae* to promote bile secretion; in cases of high fever, add *Flos Lonicerae*, *Flos Chrysanthemi Indici*, *Herba Taraxaci* and *Herba Violae* to clear away pathogenic heat.

### 3. Excess of noxious heat

Principle of treatment: Clear away heat and toxic materials. Formula of choice: Qing Dan Tang (Decoction for Clearing Away Heat from Gallbladder); in this formula, *Radix Bupleuri* regulates liver *qi* and clears away liver heat; *Radix Scutellariae, Flos Lonicerae, Herba Taraxaci* and *Fructus Forsythiae* clear away heat and eliminate toxic materials; *Radix et Rhizoma Rhei* and *Natrii Sulfas* purge excessive heat; *Fructus Aurantii Immaturus* and *Rhizoma Pinelliae* regulate and harmonize middle-*jiao*; *Radix Salviae Miltiorrhizae* nourishes blood and eliminates blood stasis.

Acupuncture treatment

Principal acupoints: Danshu (BL 19), Yanglingquan (GB 34), Taichong (LR 3), Riyue (GB 24), Qimen (LR 14), Zusanli (ST 36).

Danshu, Yanglingquan and Taichong, used together, clear away heat and regulate the flow of liver and gallbladder *qi*; Riyue and Qimen purge excessive heat in the liver and gallbladder; Zusanli replenishes the spleen and eliminates damp. Reducing method is indicated.

If there is nausea and vomiting, add Zhongwan (CV 12) and Neiguan (PC 6) to harmonize the stomach and arrest the upward adverse flow of *qi*.

If there is jaundice, add Zhiyang (GV 9) and Xingjian (LV 2) to relieve jaundice.

If there is high fever, add Quchi (LI 11), Dazhui (GV 14) and Hegu (LI 4) to clear away interior heat.

## MODERN RESEARCH

Over the past 30 years, Chinese physicians have combined traditional and Western medicines to effectively treat cholecystitis and gallstone. For example, doctors at Tianjin Nankai Hospital reported on 1,408 patients with biliary infection; 1,174 cases were successfully treated with traditional Chinese medicine, only 234 cases needed surgical intervention. This suggests that most cases of biliary infection can be cured by traditional Chinese medicine alone.

On the other hand, treating acute cholangitis of the severe type or suppurative obstructive cholecystitis or cholangitis is still a difficult problem; the mortality rate continues to be high. Hu Jiashi, et al., (Tianjin Medical College) found that combined traditional and Western medicines can have beneficial effects. They studied 38 patients with acute cholangitis of the severe type, dividing them into two groups: 20 cases in Group A received a combination of endoscopic retrograde biliary drainage (ERBD) and Decoction for Clearing Away Heat and Toxic Materials (consisting of *Herba Taraxaci, Radix Pulsatillae, Herba Patriniae, Radix Scrophulariae, Radix Glycyrrhizae* and *Radix et Rhizoma Rhei*, 15 g each, one dose per day); 18 cases in Group B received surgical drainage treatment. All 38 patients had a very high bile duct pressure (20-35 cmH$_2$O) and high levels of endotoxin in the bile and blood. The positive rate of E. coli in the bile was 84 percent. On the sixth day of treatment, the plasma bilirubin level returned to normal in 16 cases (88 percent) in Group A, but only 6 cases (33.3 percent) in group B. After operations were performed on patients in Group B, comlications of the heart, lungs or urinary tract occurred in 9 (50 percent) cases, and one patient died of multiple organ failure. Patients in Group A experienced no side effects or complications. As the authors noted, however, had the biliary obstruction not been relieved, herbal medication would have deteriorated the patients' conditions because these medications have a cholagogic action which would further increase pressure in the bile duct, thus impairing the function of the liver cells. ERBD relieved the obstruction of the bile duct, the herbal medication promoted bile drainage. Together, they reduced inflammation. On the other hand, the herbal medicines also increased the immune function and actively fought against endotoxins and bacteria.

Doctors also studied 89 patients with extrahepatic jaundice. They divided the patients into two groups randomly. Group A received choledochotomy and drainage therapy, while Group B received Li Dan Ling Decoction. Patients with incomplete biliary obstruction and those whose obstructions were relieved recovered their liver functions gradually, though the patients who had taken Li Dan Ling recovered theirs more quickly. Li Dan Ling consists of *Herba Artemisiae Capillaris* (30 g); *Radix et Rhizoma Rhei* (10 g); *Radix Glycyrrhizae* and *Radix Salviae Miltiorrhizae* (20 g each). The patients received the medication for seven-to-ten days before their operations and for two weeks afterwards.

During the last 30 years, Chinese physicians have also studied the treatment of gallstones, choledocholithiasis and postoperative residual bile duct stones. Generally speaking, if a patient is in a good condition, has no biliary stenosis and has stones less than 0.5 cm in diameter in the gallbladder or less than 1.0 cm in diameter in the common bile duct, then he is a prime candidate for treatment with traditional medicines alone or a combination of traditional and Western medicines. The most commonly used prescriptions are Yinchenhao Tang (Oriental Wormwood Decoction) and Dachaihu Tang (Major Bupleurum Decoction). In choledocholithiasis cases, the stone expulsion rate was about 60 percent, the stone evacuation rate was 30 percent, but in cholecystolithiasis evacuation rate was only 20 percent. Expelling stones usually begins on the 6th or 7th day of treatment.

In order to increase the efficacy of these medications, He Reling, et al., (Shenyang Academy of Traditional Chinese Medicine) introduced a treatment called "general attack therapy"(GAT). This method combines traditional and Western medicines for treating gallstones in the bile duct.

The protocol of GAT is as follows:

8:30 A.M. — oral administration of herbal decoction.

If the patient is in remission, the following decoction is recommended: *Herba Lysimachiae* (30 g) or *Radix Bupleuri* (9 g), *Radix Aucklandiae* (9 g), *Fructus Aurantii* (9 g), *Fructus Toosendan* (9 g), *Radix Curcumae* (12 g), *Radix Scutellariae* (6 g) and *Radix et Rhizoma Rhei* (6 g), to be prepared in decoction.

If the patient is in the attack stage, the following decoction is given: *Rhizoma Polygoni Cuspidati* and *Herba Artemisiae Scopariae* (30 g each), *Radix Aucklandiae*, *Fructus Aurantii* and *Rhizoma Corydalis* (15 g each) and *Fructus Gardeniae* (12 g), to be prepared in decoction.

9:30 A.M. — hypodermic injection of morphine, 5 mg.

10:10 A.M. — hypodermic injection of atropine, 0.5 mg.

10:15 A.M. — oral administration of 33 percent magnesium sulfate, 40 ml.

10:20 A.M. — oral administration of 5 percent diluted HCl, 30 ml.

10:25 A.M. — eating two fried eggs.

10:30 A.M. — acupuncture at right *Danshu* (BL 19).

In general, GAT is used two-to-three times per week until there is a lithagogue effect. During treatment, if the following conditions occur, surgical intervention is indicated: Aggravation of the pain, fever and jaundice; presence of peritoneal irritation; secondary pancreatitis or bile duct bleeding; failure to repond to GAT. According to report by He Reling, et al., among 91 patients with residual extra- and intrahepatic choledocholithiasis treated with GAT, 55 (60.4 percent) experienced expulsion of stones and 18 (33 percent) evacuation of stones, as determined by cholangiography.

# CHAPTER XIII    ULCERATIVE COLITIS

Ulcerative colitis is a chronic disease of unknown etiology characterized by inflammation of the mucosa and submucosa of the large intestine. The inflammation usually involves the rectum and the anal margin and extends proximally in the colon for a variable distance.

The five most common symtoms of ulcerative colitis are rectal bleeding, diarrhea, abdominal pain, weight loss and fever. The disease may begin in a subtle manner or with catastrophic suddenness. Patients may relate the acute onset of symptoms to a recent emotional upset, to an upper respiratory infection or to oral antibiotic therapy.

The diagnosis of ulcerative colitis is based on its clinical manifestations, demonstration of inflammation of the rectal and sigmoidal mucosa using proctosigmoidoscopy, identification of specific infections through appropriate stool cultures and examination for parasites. The diagnosis may be supported by radiologic examination, colonoscopy and rectal biopsy.

In traditional Chinese medicine, ulcerative colitis is associated with syndromes of "diarrhea," "abdominal pain," and "bloody stool."

## ETIOLOGY AND PATHOGENESIS

1. Deficiency of the spleen fails to keep blood flowing within the vessels, leading to bloody stool. Protracted deficiency of the spleen may attack the kidneys, resulting in deficiency of both the spleen and kidneys. On the other hand, deficiency of the spleen also may cause damp to accumulate in the large intestine.

2. Excessive intake of pungent and greasy food or alcoholic drink causes damp-heat to accumulate in the lower-*jiao* and damage the intestinal collaterals.

3. Emotional upset and rage cause liver *qi* to stagnate, which adversely attacks the spleen, resulting in incoordination between the liver and spleen.

## DIFFERENTIAL DIAGNOSIS OF SYNDROMES

### 1. Deficiency of the spleen
Primary manifestations: Loose and mucopurulent bloody stool, lower abdominal distension or discomfort, sallow complexion, poor appetite, weight loss, pale tongue with deep and small pulse.

### 2. Accumulation of damp-heat in the middle-*jiao*
Primary manifestations: Loose and mucopurulent bloody stool, lower abdominal pain and tenderness, low-grade fever, thirst with preference for cold drink, reddened tongue with yellow, greasy coating and rapid pulse.

93

### 3. Attack of the stagnated liver *qi* on the spleen

Primary manifestations: Diarrhea with mucopurulent bloody stool, hypochondriac distension, nausea, irritability, thirst with bitter taste in the mouth, slightly reddened tongue with thin coating and taut pulse.

## TREATMENT

### 1. Deficiency of the spleen

Principle of treatment: Replenish *qi* and strengthen the spleen.

Formula of choice: Guipi Tang (Decoction for Invigorating the Spleen and Nourishing the Heart) and Shen Ling Baizhu San (Powder of Ginseng, Poria and White Atractylodes); in these prescriptions, *Radix Genseng*, Poria, *Rhizoma Atractylodis Macrocephalae*, *Radix Glycyrrhizae*, *Radix Astragali*, *Semen Dolichoris Album*, *Rhizoma Dioscoreae*, *Semen Nelumbinis* and *Semen Coicis* replenish the spleen and strengthen middle-*qi*; *Radix Angelicae Sinensis* nourishes the blood; *Radix Aucklandiae* and *Fructus Amomi* regulate *qi* and harmonize the stomach; other ingredients listed in these prescriptions may be omitted; patients with *yang* deficiency of both the spleen and kidneys manifested by cold limbs, pallor, lassitude and diarrhea occurring before dawn daily should receive Sishen Wan (Pill of Four Miraculous Drugs) and Huangtu Tang (Decoction of Baked Yellow Earth); in these formulae, *Fructus Psoraleae* replenishes fire in the vital gate; *Radix Aconiti Praeparata*, *Fructus Evodiae* and baked Ginger warm the middle-*jiao* and expel cold; *Semen Myristicae* and *Fructus Schisandrae* are astringents for relieving diarrhea; *Radix Rehmanniae* and *Colla Corii Asini* nourish blood; Baked Yellow Earth stops bleeding; and *Radix Scutellariae* protects the blood from being damaged by drugs that are warm in nature.

### 2. Accumulation of damp-heat in the middle-*jiao*

Principle of treatment: Clear away damp heat.

Formula of choice: Diyu San (Powder of *Radix Sanguisorbae*) and Chixiaodou Danggui San (Powder of Phaseolus Seeds and Chinese Angelica Root); in these prescriptions, *Radix Sanguisorbae* and *Radix Rubiae* clear away heat from the blood and stop bleeding; *Radix Angelicae Sinensis* nourishes blood; *Radix Scutellariae*, *Rhizoma Coptidis* and *Fructus Gardeniae*, bitter in taste and cool in nature, clear away heat and remove damp; Poria and *Semen Phaseoli* replenish the spleen and remove the damp; if the patient has a greasy tongue coating or fever, add *Herb Agastachis* and *Herba Eupatorii* to relieve exterior syndrome and expel damp.

### 3. Attack of stagnated liver *qi* on the spleen

Principle of treatment: Regulate liver *qi* and strengthen the spleen.

Formula of choice: Tongxie Yaofang (Prescription of Importance for Diarrhea with Pain); in this prescription, *Rhizoma Atractylodis Macrocephalae* replenishes the spleen; *Radix Paeoniae Alba* nourishes blood and harmonizes the liver; *Pericarpium Citri Reticulatae* regulates middle *qi*; *Radix Saposhinkoviae* regulates liver *qi*; if there is marked rectal bleeding, add *Flos Sophorae Immaturus*, *Radix Sanguisorbae*, *Radix Notoginseng* Powder, *Rhizoma Blelillae* and *Herba Agrimoniae*.

Acupuncture treatment

Principal points: Zhongwan (CV 12), Tianshu (ST 25), Zusanli (ST 36) and Qihai (CV 6) are selected for needling or moxibustion to regulate the function of the stomach and intestines.

Supplementary points:

1. For deficiency of the spleen, add Pishu (BL 20) and Taibai (SP 3) to strengthen the function of the spleen in transporting and transforming and to stop diarrhea.

2. For deficiency of the kidneys, add Shenshu (BL 23), Mingmen (GV 4), Guanyan (CV 4) and Taixi (KI 3) to reinforce the fire of the vital gate, strengthen the kidneys and promote digestion.

3. For stagnation of liver *qi*, add Qimen (LR 14) and Taichong (LR 3) to regulate the flow of *qi*, remove stagnated liver *qi* and stop diarrhea.

# MODERN RESEARCH

Form 1975 to 1987, physicians studied 1,830 cases of ulcerative colitis treated with traditional Chinese medicine. The total effective rate among these patients was 95.2 percent — 62.6 percent were cured and 32.6 percent improved. Doctors also found that contrary to oral herbal medications, retention enemas with herbal medicines produced more marked results. They recommended the following enteroclysis prescriptions:

1. Enema with sterilized radish juice (100-200 ml), once daily.

2. *Herba Portulacae* (50 g), *Radix Pulsatillae* (50 g) and *Cortex Phellodendri* (50 g) made into a 100 ml decoction and add 20 ml of 2% procaine, administer enema once daily.

3. *Radix Sophorae Flavescentis* (30 g), *Cortex Ailanthi* (30 g), *Radix Pulsatillae* (30 g), *Radix Arnebiae seu Lithospermi* (30 g) and *Rhizoma Coptidis* (10 g) made into a 200 ml decoction; administer 50-100 ml enema, twice daily.

4. Alumen (9 g), *Radix et Rhizoma Rhei* (6 g), *Rhizoma Atractylodis* (9 g), *Radix Sophorae Elavescentis* (9 g) and *Flos Sophorae* (9 g) made into a 200 ml decoction; administer 50-100 ml enema, twice daily.

5. *Radix Pulsatillae* (15 g), *Cortex Phellodendri* (15 g), *Rhizoma Atractylodis* (10 g), *Rhizoma Polygoni Cuspidati* (10 g), *Radix Angelicae Sinensis* (10 g), *Rhizoma Ligustici* (10 g), *Radix Paeoniae Alba* (10 g) and *Fructus Aurantii* (10 g) made into a 200 ml decoction; administer 50-100 ml enema, twice daily.

The above-mentioned treatment may be used in combination with Western medicines in severe cases.

# CHAPTER XIV    ACUTE PANCREATITIS

The pathogenesis of pancreatitis remains obscure. Therefore, treatment with Western medicine is supportive rather than specific.

Pancreatitis is either acute or chronic. An attack of pancreatitis is defined as acute if the patient becomes asymptomatic following recovery. The hallmark of acute pancreatitis is abdominal pain. In chronic pancreatitis, the patient has persistent pain or insufficient exocrine or endocrine pancreatic secretion.

## ETIOLOGY AND PATHOGENESIS

In traditional Chinese medicine, the pancreas' function is related to those of the ‣spleen and stomach as well as the liver and gallbladder. Therefore, the pathogenesis of acute pancreatitis is associated with the dysfunction of the spleen, stomach, liver and gallbladder. The basic pathological condition is a syndrome of excess, heat and interior. It relates to the following factors:

1. Emotional upset stagnates liver *qi*, which disrupts its flow and interferes with the secretion of bile.

2. Overeating greasy food or drinking excessive amounts of alcohol causes damp-heat to accumulate in the middle-*jiao*, which steams the liver and gallbladder and disturbs the *qi* of the *fu*-organs. Either stagnation of liver *qi* or accumulation of damp-heat in the middle-*jiao* may cause blood stasis.

3. Excessive pathogenic damp-heat rapidly penetrating into the interior damages the pericardium, disturbing consciousness.

## DIFFERENTIAL DIAGNOSIS OF SYNDROMES

### 1. Stagnation of liver *qi*
Primary manifestations: Abdominal pain often localized to the epigastrium and left upper quadrant, nausea and vomiting, abdominal distension or bilateral hypochondriac distending pain, eructation, low fever, thin and white tongue coating and taut pulse (Acute pancreatitis with mild interstitial edema shares these manifestations).

### 2. Accumulation of damp-heat in the spleen and stomach
Primary manifestations: Severe abdominal pain often localized to the epigastrium and left upper quadrant and aggravated by pressure, high fever, nausea, vomiting, thirst without preference for beverages, reddened tongue with yellow and greasy coating and rapid pulse.

### 3. Attack of excessive damp-heat on the pericardium
Primary manifestations: High fever, abdominal pain in the epigastrium and left upper abdomen with tenderness or diffuse abdominal pain radiating to the back,

spontaneous sweating, pale complexion, shortness of breath, cold limbs, lassitude, reddened tongue with yellow, greasy coating and thready and rapid pulse (Hemorrhagic and necrotic pancreatitis shares these manifestations).

# TREATMENT

Principle of treatment: Regulate liver *qi*, purge heat, eliminate damp and remove blood stasis.

Formula of choice: Formulae are based on Da Chaihu Tang (Major Bupleurum Decoction), Chaihu Shugan San (Bupleurum Powder for Relieving Liver *Qi*) and Huanglian Jiedu Tang (Antidotal Decoction of Coptis).

Doctors at Tianjin Nankai Hospital developed a basic prescription for treating various types of acute pancreatitis called Decoction No. 1 for Treating Acute Pancreatitis. In this prescription, *Radix Bupleuri* and *Radix Aucklandiae* regulate liver *qi*; *Rhizoma Coptidis* and *Radix Scutellariae* remove damp and clear away heat; *Radix Paeoniae Alba* and *Rhizoma Corydalis* promote blood circulation and remove blood stasis; and *Radix et Rhizoma Rhei* and *Natrii Sulfas* purge interior heat and toxic materials. Modifications to this formula are as follows:

In case of excessive heat, add *Flos Lonicerae* and *Fructus Forsythiae*.

In case of excessive damp-heat, add *Fructus Gardeniae, Herba Artemisiae Capillaris* and *Rhizoma Alismatis.*

In case of obstruction of biliary duct by ascarid, add *Semen Arecae, Fructus Quisqualis, Cortex Meliae* and *Herba Asari.*

In case of spontaneous sweating, pale complexion, shortness of breath, thready and rapid pulse, treatment of shock is necessary. Since acute hemorrhagic necrotic pancreatitis is a serious condition with a high mortality rate, combined treatment of Western and traditional Chinese medicines is recommended.

Acupuncture Treatment

Main acupoints: Shangwan (CV 13), Neiguan (PC 6), Zusanli (ST 36) and Yanglingquan (GB 34).

Modifications:

If there is abdominal distention, add Tianshu (ST 25) and Qihai (CV 6).

If there is fever, add Quchi (LI 11) and Hegu (LI 4).

If there is jaundice, add Danshu (BL 19) and Qiuxu (GB 40).

If there is hypotension, add Renzhong (GV 26) and Baihui (GV 20).

If there is excessive damp-heat, add Waiguan (TE 5), Taichong (LR 3) and Yinlingquan (SP 9).

# MODERN RESEARCH

Medical treatment of acute pancreatitis in Western medicine is largely symptomatic and supportive. The average mortality is about 10 percent.

Over the past 30 years, physicians have used traditional Chinese medicine to treat acute pancreatitis in China. In mild and moderately severe cases, more than 90 percent were cured, and the mortality rate was between one and two percent. This traditional approach differs from Western medicine in that starvation and gastric suction are usually not necessary, nor is the prophylactic use of antibiotics.

Hemorrhagic pancreatitis is another matter and should be treated with combined traditional and Western medicines. In the early stage of hemorrhagic pancreatitis, most patients have a complicated syndrome of deficiency and excess, i.e., the body resistance is weakened while pathogenic factors prevail. Therefore, treatment is aimed at strengthening the body resistance to eliminate pathogenic factors. The principal prescription is Shengmai San (Pulse-Activating Powder), in addition to Decoction No. 1 for Treating Acute Pancreatitis. Pulse-Activating Powder replenishes *qi*, nourishes *yin*, stops sweating and cures collapse (prostration). Wang Baoen, et al., (Beijing Friendship Hospital) reported on 29 cases of acute hemorrhagic necrotic pancreatitis treated with combined herbal and Western medicines, including antibiotics. "Purgation" was the main purpose of the treatments used and Rhubarb was the chief ingredient. Formulae included:

1. Major Bupleurum Decoction:

2. Decoction for Purging Heat, consisting of Rhubarb (30 g), *Natrii Sulfas* (10 g), Scrophularia (15 g) and Liquorice (6 g) made into a 200 ml decoction, taken orally 3-4 times daily in 50-100 ml dosages.

3. Rhubarb (30 g) made into a 200 ml decoction taken orally 3-4 times daily in 50-100 ml doses.

All these prescriptions contain Rhubarb to purge heat. When mild diarrhea occurs, these purgative decoctions should be stopped.

Wang Baoen reported that among the 29 cases, 27 were cured and only two died, the mortality rate being 6.9 percent. Wang and his fellow researchers contend that herbal medications played an important role in lowering the mortality rate.

Ren Shiguang, et al., (Beijing Friendship Hospital) observed the role of virus in hemorrhagic pancreatitis and the therapeutic effect of Rhubarb. Ren and his assoociates injected live measles vaccine into the main pancreatic duct and the ear vein of rabbits. The level of serum amylase was significantly higher than that of the rabbits injected with saline. The platelet aggregation also increased, and the doctors observed congestion and hemorrhage of the pancreas. They divided rabbits with experimental pancreatitis into two groups. The group treated with Rhubarb experienced a reduction in serum amylase that surpassed that of the control group. Platelet aggregation was also inhibited, congestion and hemorrhage of the pancreas were less obvious. In addition to the effectiveness of Rhubarb in treating hemorrhagic pancreatitis, this research suggests that virus might be one of the pathogenic factors which causes this disease.

Chen, et al., observed the effect of Ginseng in rats with acute experimental hemorrhagic pancreatitis induced by injecting sodium taurocholate into their pancreatic ducts. The mortality rate in the control group was 75 percent, 40 percent in the Ginseng group. Reduction of blood flow, hemorrhage and necrosis as well as damage of the mitochondria in the pancreas were less marked in the Ginseng group than in the control group. Ginseng also lowered the level of plasma amylase.

Kong Li, et al., (Tianjin Nankai Hospital) studied the action of Qing Yi Injection on pancreatic exocrine and its ability to protect against caerulein-induced acute experimental pancreatitis in rats. Qing Yi Injection consists of *Radix Bupleuri, Radix Scutellariae, Rhizoma Picrorrhizae, Radix Inulae, Pericarpium Arecae, Radix Aucklandiae* and *Radix Glycyrrhizae.*

Results of the study showed that Qing Yi Injection promoted the delivery of pancreatic juice and amylase and reduced the amylase activity in the serum and pancreas. It provided protection against caerulein-induced pancreatitis, which may be attributed to its stimulation of pancreatic exocrine and inhibition of pancreatic enzymes. It had no effect on phospholipase A.

Wang Guixi, et al., (Sun Yat-sen Medical University, Guangzhou) observed the effect of electroacupuncture of the Zusanli (ST 36) acupoint on exocrine secretion of pancreas in rats. The study indicated that electroacupuncture could inhibit protein secretion in both conscious and anesthetized rats. The authors believe that this inhibiting mechanism may be similar to the effect Qing Yi Injection has on protein (enzyme) secretion of the pancreas.

Respiratory depression syndrome (RDS) is one of the main causes of death in acute hemorrhagic necrotic pancreatitis. Zheng Shusen, et al., (First Teaching Hospital, West China Medical University, Chengdu) studied the protective effects of Salvia militiorrhiza on early lung injuries in acute hemorrhagic necrotic pancreatitis in dogs. Zheng and his associates experimentally induced acute hemorrhagic necrotic pancreatitis in 18 healthy adult dogs of both sexes by retrograde injection of sodium taurocholate directly into their pancreatic ducts. The authors treated one group of dogs with intravenous infusions of *Radix Salviae Miltiorrhizae* (5 g/kg), and the other group with Anisodamine 654-2 (5 mg/kg) or normal saline. The lactic acid dehydrogenase (LDH), albumin and lipid peroxide (LPO) levels in the bronchoalveolar lavage fluid were significantly higher in the dogs who received the saline treatment compared with those of the Salvia miltiorrhiza group ($P < 0.05$). The doctors observed necrosis and disruption of conjunction of the endothelial cells resulting from defects in the vascular wall under transmission electron microscope. They found that both pulmonary vascular and type II pneumocytes were normal in the Salvia miltiorrhiza group, suggesting that Salvia miltiorrhiza can protect endothelial cells of the pulmonary vessels and type II pneumocytes.

# CHAPTER XV    VIRAL HEPATITIS

Viral hepatitis is caused by hepatitis viruses A and B and the so called "non-A non-B" agents. The earliest symptoms of acute viral hepatitis are nonspecific, predominantly constitutional and gastrointestinal. They may include malaise, fatigue, anorexia, nausea, vomiting, jaundice and pain in the liver area. Fever, if present, is usually mild. A sustained inflammatory process in the liver lasting more than six months is considered chronic hepatitis. In most cases, hepatocellular necrosis occurs. Most chronic viral hepatitis is caused by hepatitis B and non-A non-B viruses. The course of chronic hepatitis may vary greatly. Patients may be asymptomatic or exhibit a wide range of local or constitutional symptoms. Based on its symptoms, viral hepatitis is associated with "jaundice," "hypochondrium pain," "stagnation syndrome," "vomiting" and "abdominal mass" in traditional Chinese medicine.

## ETIOLOGY AND PATHOGENESIS

Epidemic pathogens or pathogenic damp-heat accumulated in the interior of the body cause viral hepatitis.

1. Epidemic pathogens infect the liver and gallbladder, which results in heat or damp-heat that affects the smooth flow of liver *qi* and secretion of bile and leads to jaundice, anorexia and malaise.

2. Improper diet or abnormal weather causes dysfunction of the spleen in transportation and transformation, leading to retention of damp-heat in the spleen and stomach which further injures the liver and gallbladder.

3. Exuberant pathogenic damp-heat accumulated in the interior of the body for a long time impairs vital essence; as a result, deficiency of *yin, yang, qi* or blood syndromes may occur. In serious cases, epidemic pathogens or damp-heat may invade the pericardium and cause coma or other central nervous symptoms.

## DIFFERENTIAL DIAGNOSIS OF SYNDROMES

1. Differentiation of *yang*-jaundice versus *yin*-jaundice: Affection due to damp-heat is known as *yang* jaundice. It is characterized by a lustrous yellow discoloration of the skin and sclera, fever, anorexia, nausea, dryness and bitter taste in the mouth, pain in the right hypochondriac region, yellow, greasy tongue coating and taut, slippery and rapid pulse. Affection due to cold-dampness is known as *yin* jaundice and is marked by dark yellow discoloration of sclera and smoky-coloured skin, lassitude, poor appetite, pale tongue with thick, greasy coating and deep, small and weak or slow pulse. *Yang* jaundice is commonly seen in acute viral hepatitis, *yin* jaundice in chronic hepatitis.

2. Determination of preponderance of heat over damp or vice versa: Damp-heat is

the most common pathogenic factor in jaundice. However, damp-heat invades the body in different ways, so that some patients have a preponderance of heat symptoms and others a preponderance of damp symptoms. Fever, thirst, constipation, scanty dark yellow urine, reddened tongue with yellow coating and rapid pulse mark cases of preponderant heat. Cases of preponderant damp, on the other hand, are characterized by a heavy sensation of the body, anorexia, nausea, fullness in the abdomen, stuffiness of the chest, loose stool, whitish, thick and greasy tongue coating and slippery pulse.

In protracted cases, pathogenic damp-heat may consume *yin* of the liver and kidneys, leading to *yin* deficiency of both viscera. The symtoms of this condition are feverish sensation in the palms, thirst, dizziness, tinnitus, insomnia, lumbago, weakness of the legs, reddened tongue with little or no coating and fine and rapid pulse (in addition to the general clinical manifestations of damp-heat).

3. Recognition of deficiency versus excess: Most acute hepatitis cases are of the excess type, while a majority of chronic hepatitis patients are in a condition of deficiency and excess, manifested as weakness, lassitude, poor appetite, nausea and loose stool. In some cases, exuberant damp-heat remains in the interior of the body or virulent epidemic pathogens affect the body with the result that the pericardium is attacked and *yin*-blood consumed. This condition is marked by fever, progressive jaundice, fetor hepaticus, restlessness, delirium, epistaxis, odontorrhagia, hematemesis, distension and fullness in the abdomen, oliguria, edema, ascites and even hepatic coma. The tongue is usually dry and reddened, covered with a yellow, greasy coating, and the pulse is small, weak and rapid. This syndrome is usually seen in fulminat hepatitis or subacute hepatic necrosis.

4. Determination of stagnation of *qi* versus blood stasis: In the early stage of the disease, liver *qi* stagnates, which affects the function of the spleen and stomach and leads to a disturbance between the liver and stomach manifested as anorexia, abdominal distention, hypochondriac pain varying with emotional changes and irritability. In some cases, stagnated liver *qi* leads to blood stasis, manifested as hepatomegaly with stabbing pain, tenderness, dark purplish complexion, vascular spider and petechiae or ecchymoses (in addition to the manifestations of stagnation of liver *qi*). Stagnated liver *qi* may cause dysfunction of the spleen in transporting and transforming, thus causing water to accumulate. In addition, blood stasis may also disturb water metabolism and consequently cause edema and ascites.

## TREATMENT

### 1. Clear away damp heat

If heat is preponderant, Yinchenhao Tang (Oriental Wormwood Decoction) is used to clear away damp-heat. *Rhizoma Polyani*, *Radix Scutellariae*, *Flos Chrysanthemi Indici*, *Rhizoma Smilacis Glabrae* and *Radix Isatidis* can be added to strengthen the effect of this formula. For fever, *Radix Bupleuri*, *Radix Scutellariae* and *Radix Isatidis* may be added to clear away the heat. Adding *Radix Paeoniae Rubra* will cool and activate the blood. For severe nausea or vomiting, *Rhizoma Pinelliae* and *Caulis Bambusae in Taeniam* should be added to harmonize the stomach and keep its *qi* flowing downwards. For pain in the right hypochondriac area, add *Radix Curcumae* and *Fructus*

*Mediae Toosendau* to regulate the flow of the stagnated liver *qi* and ease pain. For anorexia, administer *Massa Fermentata Medicinalis*, *Fructus Aurantii Immaturus* and *Fructus Crataegi* to regulate *qi* and whet the appetite.

If damp is preponderant, Yinchen Wuling San (Powder of Oriental Wormwood and Five Drugs with Poria) is the formula of choice. The *Herba Artemisiae Scopariae* in this prescription eliminates damp and increases secretion of bile; the other ingredients invigorate the spleen and eliminate damp.

### 2. Warm the middle-*jiao* and eliminating damp

Yinchen Zhu Fu Tang (Decoction of Oriental Wormwood, White Atractylodes and Aconite) is used to treat *yin* jaundice. In this formula, *Herba Artemisiae Scopariae* and *Radix Aconiti Lateralis Praeparata* expel cold-damp; *Rhizoma Atractylodis Macrocephalae, Radix Zingiberis Praeparata* and *Radix Glycyrrhizae* warm the middle-*jiao* and invigorate the spleen; and Poria and *Rhizoma Alismatis* eliminate damp. For cases with deficiency of the spleen, add *Radix Codonopsis Pilosulae* and *Radix Astragali* to replenish *qi* of the middle-*jiao*.

### 3. Relieve depressed liver *qi* and invigorate the spleen

Chaihu Shugan San (Bupleurum Powder for Relieving Depressed Liver *Qi*) and Si Junzi Tang (Decoction of Four Noble Drugs) invigorate the spleen and replenish *qi*.

### 4. Nourish *yin* of the liver and kidneys

For *yin* deficiency of the liver and kidneys, Yiguan Jian (Ever-effective Decoction for Nourishing the Liver and Kidneys) is used to treat *yin* deficiency of the liver and kidneys. In this prescription, *Radix Adenophorae Strictae, Radix Ophiopogonis, Radix Angelicae Sinensis, Radix Rehmanniae* and *Fructus Lycii* nourish liver and kidney *yin*, and *Fructus Meliae Toosendan* regulates liver *qi*. For cases with afternoon fever, add *Cortex Moutan Radicis, Cortex Lycii Radicis* and *Herba Artemisiae Scopariae* to expel heat due to *yin* deficiency. For cases with thirst and poor appetite, add *Herba Dendrobii, Fructus Crataegi* and *Endothelium Corneum Gigeriae Galli* to strengthen production of body fluids and improve the appetite.

### 5. Regulate liver *qi* and remove blood stasis

Xuefu Zhuyu Tang (Decoction for Removing Blood Stasis in the Chest) is used to treat stagnated liver *qi* and blood stasis. In this prescription, *Radix Angelicae Sinensis, Radix Rehmanniae, Semen Persicae, Flos Carthami, Radix Paeoniae Rubra* and *Rhizoma Ligustici Chuanxiong* promote blood circulation and remove blood stasis. *Radix Bupleuri* and *Fructus Aurantii* regulate liver *qi*. *Radix Glycyrrhizae* harmonizes the middle-*jiao* and coordinates the actions of the other ingredients in the prescription. *Radix Platycodi* acts as a guide drug.

In severe cases, when pathogenic heat invades the blood system causing high fever, eruptions and hemorrhages, Xijiao Dihuang Tang (Decoction Rhinoceros Horn and Rehmannia) is adopted with modifications. In this prescription, *Cornu Rhinoceri* cools the blood and expels toxic materials; *Radix Rehmanniae, Radix Paeoniae Rubra* and *Cortex Moutan Radicis* cool the blood, clear away heat and remove blood stasis.

The therapies described above can be used individually or in combination. Acute or subacute hepatic necrosis requires combined traditional Chinese and Western medicines.

Acupuncture treatment

Principal points: Insert needles at Ganshu (BL 18), Danshu (BL 19), Pishu (BL 20), Zusanli (ST 36) and Zhiyang (GV 9) points to regulate the flow of *qi* in the liver and gallbladder and strengthen the function of the spleen.

Supplementary points:

1. For cases with accumulation of damp-heat, add Yanglingquan (GB 34), Taichong (LR 3), Dazhui (GV 14) and Jianshi (PC 5) to eliminate damp-heat from the liver and gallbladder.

2. For cases with accumulation of cold-damp, perform needling and moxibustion at Yanggang (BL 48), Yinlingquan (SP 9) and Sanyinjiao (SP 6) to warm the spleen and eliminate dampness.

3. For cases with deficiency of *yin*, add Taichong (LR 3) and Taixi (KI 3) to nourish *yin* of the liver and kidneys.

4. For cases with stagnation of *qi* and blood stasis, add Taichong (LR 3), Qiuxu (GB 40) and Geshu (BL 17) to regulate liver and gallbladder *qi*, promote blood circulation and remove stasis.

# MODERN RESEARCH

In general, patients with excess syndrome usually have mild hepatopathologic lesions (an inflammatory reaction), degeneration of liver cells and infiltration of inflammatory cells. In cases with deficiency syndrome, patients experience a variety of necrosis and fibrosis in the liver. Stasis of hepatic sinusoid, lobular disruption and fibrosis are often found in cases with blood stasis.

Because acute viral hepatitis is a self-limited disease, we have only considered traditional Chinese treatments of chronic viral hepatitis here. Several studies of the clinical effective rate of traditional Chinese medicine on chronic viral hepatitis based on differentiation of syndromes indicated a range of effectiveness between 70 and 93.3 percent; the negative-conversion rates of HBsAg, HBeAg and HBV-DNA were 40-to-50 percent in HBV-carriers.

Han Jinghuan, et al., (Shanxi Provincial Institute of Traditional Chinese Medicine, Taiyuan) observed the therapeutic effects of No. 1 and No. 2 Decoctions to Replenish the Liver on chronic hepatitis. Of 358 patients, 204 with deficiency syndrome received Decoction No. 1, 154 with excess syndrome received Decoction No. 2. (Decoction No. 1 consists of *Radix Codonopsis Pilosulae*, *Radix Astragali*, Poria, *Rhizoma Atractylodis Macrocephalae*, *Radix Glycyrrhizae*, *Radix Angelicae Sinensis*, *Radix Rehmanniae*, *Radix Salviae Miltiorrhizae*, *Radix Curcumae*, *Herba Artemisiae Scopariae*, *Radix Isatidis*, *Rhizoma Alismatis*, *Fructus Crataegi* and *Rhizoma Dioscoreae*; Decoction No. 2 consists of *Flos Lonicerae*, *Herba Patriniae*, *Radix Gentianae*, *Fructus Gardeniae*, *Radix Salviae Miltiorrhizae*, *Radix Angelicae Sinensis*, *Radix Paeoniae*, *Radix Codonopsis Pilosulae*, *Rhizoma Atractylodis Macrocephalae*, Poria, *Radix Curcumae*, *Herba Artemisiae Scopariae*, *Semen Plantaginis*, *Fructus Citri*, *Radix Glycyrrhizae* and *Semen Raphani*.) Patients received one dose orally each day for four-to-six months. The short-term clinical cure rate of those patients who had received Decoction No. 1 was 86.3 percent and 79.9 percent for those who'd received Decoction No. 2. Liver function returned to normal in 87.3 percent of the former and 80.5 percent of the latter. The actions of these formulae included protecting liver cells, accelerating the generation of hepatocytes, inhibiting hepatic fibrosis, regulating immunological responses, improving microcirculation and increasing the secretion of bile.

Wu Weiyi, et al., reported on 326 cases of chronic hepatitis treated with glycyrrhizic acid, a substance extracted from *Radix Glycyrrhizae*. The total effective rate observed was 86.5 percent. Treatment was characterized by rapid relief of symptoms, such as jaundice and abnormal GPT and GOT levels, but no change in protein-regulation and HBV-marker.

In a related study, doctors used diphenyldiester, a substance extracted from *Fructus Schisandrae*, to reduce elevated plasma transaminase and achieved an effective rate of 90 percent. However, this substance sometimes exacerbated the disease, a complication which stopped as soon as the drug was no longer administered.

Wang, et al., compared the effects of combined therapy with Western therapy alone on 215 patients suffering from subacute severe hepatitis. Group A (169 patients) received *Herba Artemisiae Scopariae, Fructus Gardeniae* and *Radix Scutellariae* Injections (AGSI) and Compound Decoction of Rhubarb (CDR) in combination with Western medicine. Group B (46 patients) received only Western medicine. The clinical conditions of the two groups were comparable. The mortality rate was 70.4 percent in Group A and 89.1 percent in Group B. The study revealed that AGSI and CDR could promote the production of interferon induced by virus. As a result, interferon levels increased by twice those of normal. During corticosteroid treatment, the incidence of complicating infections was 7.7 percent in Group A and 24.5 percent in Group B.

# CHAPTER XVI   APLASTIC ANEMIA

Aplastic anemia includes a diverse group of potentially severe bone marrow disorders. Some are characterized by periperal pancytopenia, in which large amounts of fat replace hematopoietic cells in the marrow while the bone retains its basic architecture or stroma. Other disorders manifest unicellular aplasia, i.e., pure red cell aplasia.

In approximately 50 percent of aplastic anemia cases the cause is unknown, and the anemia is considered idiopathic. The other 50 percent of cases are associated with exposure to an array of chemicals or ionizing radiation, or with contraction of neoplastic, autoimmune or infectious diseases. Few clinical differences exist between the idiopathic and secondary forms of the disease. The onset of aplastic anemia is usually insidious but may be dramatic. Bleeding is typically the first manifestation. Gingival bleeding, epistaxis and petechiae are commonly seen; they are often related to severe thrombocytopenia. Fatigue, pallor and various infections often occur in severe cases.

Traditional Chinese medicine classifies aplastic anemia as a syndrome of consumption or of blood deficiency.

## ETIOLOGY AND PATHOGENESIS

### 1. Damage of the marrow by virulent heat
Aplastic anemia may occur when virulent heat attacks the marrow.
### 2. Deficiency of spleen *qi*
The spleen produces blood by transforming the food essence. Furthermore, spleen *qi* keeps blood circulating in the vessels and prevents bleeding. If spleen *qi* is insufficient and fails to promote the normal transporting and transforming of food, the refined substances required for producing blood and controlling circulation will be insufficient and eventually lead to anemia and bleeding.
### 3. Deficiency of liver and kidney *yin*
The kidneys store vital essence which may be transformed into blood, and dominate the regeneration of bone marrow. The liver stores blood. Therefore, deficiency of *yin* (essential substances) of the liver and kidneys is one of the basic pathogenic factors of aplastic anemia.

## DIFFERENTIAL DIAGNOSIS OF SYNDROMES

The Hematological Society, part of the Chinese Association for the Integration of Traditional and Western Medicine, recommended the following classifications of syndrome patterns in aplastic anemia in 1982.
### 1. Damage of marrow by virulent heat
Primary manifestations: Abrupt onset, pallor or sallow complexion, general lassitude,

fever, dizziness, palpitations, shortness of breath, petechiae, epistasis or menorrhagia, delirium and coma in severe cases, pale tongue with yellowish white and greasy coating and weak and rapid pulse.

This pattern often occurs in acute aplastic anemia caused by virulent heat.

**2. *Yang* deficiency in the spleen and kidneys**

Primary manifestations: Pallor or sallow complexion, general lassitude, aversion to cold, cold limbs, soreness and weakness of the lower back and knees, spontaneous sweating, poor appetite, abdomenal distention, puffiness of the face or edema of the lower extremities, petechiae, epistaxis or menorrhagia, pale tongue with white coating and thready and weak pulse.

**3. *Yin* deficiency in the liver and kidneys**

Primary manifestations: General lassitude, dizziness, ringing in the ears, insomnia, amnesia, dry mouth and throat, feverish sensation in the palms, soles and chest, petechiae epitaxis or menorrhagia, lack of saliva, thin and yellow tongue coating and thready and rapid pulse.

**4. Deficiency of both *yin* and *yang* in the kidneys**

Primary manifestations: Pallor or sallow complexion, general lassitude, palpitations, shortness of breath, soreness and weakness of the lower back and knees, spontaneous sweating, cold limbs, restlessness, insomnia, dry mouth and throat, dizziness, petechiae, epistaxis, menorrhagia, lack of saliva, white tongue coating or absence of coating and thready, rapid and weak pulse.

The latter three patterns often occur in chronic aplastic anemia.

## TREATMENT

**1. Acute marrow consumption by virulent heat**

Principle of treatment: cool blood and expel virulent heat.

Formula of choice: Qingwen Baidu Yin (Antipyretic and Antitoxic Decoction) with modifications, including: Baihu Tang (White Tiger Decoction), which clears away heat and promotes production of body fluids; Xijiao Dihuang Tang (Decoction of Rhinoceros Horn and Rehmannia), which clears away heat and toxic materials, cools the blood and removes blood stasis; and Huanglian Jiedu Tang (Antidotal Decoction of Coptis), which purges the pathogenic fire and heat in the triple-*jiao*.

**2. *Yang* deficiency in the spleen and kidneys**

Principle of treatment: warm and invigorate both *yang* of the spleen and kidneys.

Formula of choice: Yougui Wan (Kidney-*yang* Reinforcing Bolus) and Buzhong Yiqi Tang (Docoction for Reinforcing Middle-*jiao* and Replenishing *qi*); Yougui Wan warms *yang* and invigorates the kidneys; *Radix Rehmanniae Praeparatae, Fructus Corni, Fructus Lycii* and *Radix Angelicae Sinensis* in this formula replenish and nourish liver and kidney *yin, Radix Aconiti Praeparata* and *Cortex Cinnamomi* warm and replenish kidney *yang* and *Cortex Eucommiae, Semen Cuscutae* and *Colla Cornus Cervi* strengthen the kidneys and nourish vital essence.

**3. *Yin* deficiency of the liver and kidneys**

Principle of treatment: nourish *yin* of the liver and kidneys.

Formula of choice: Zuogui Wan (Kidney-*yin* Replenishing Bolus) and Siwu Tang (Decoction of Four Ingredients); the following ingredients are included in these formulae: *Fructus Lycii, Radix Rehmanniae Praeparata, Fructus Corni* and *Colla Plastri Testudinis* nourish *yin* of the liver and kidneys; *Radix Angelicae Sinensis* and *Radix Paeoniae Alba* nourish liver blood; Poria, *Rhizoma Dioscoreae* and *Radix Glycyrrhizae Praeparata* nourish *yin* of the liver and kidneys by stimulating the function of the spleen; and *Radix Ginseng* and *Radix Astragali* replenish *qi* and promote the production of *yin*.

**4. Deficiency of *yin* and *yang* in the kidneys**
Principle of treatment: replenish *yin* and *yang* of the kidneys.

Formula of choice: Zuogui Wan and Yougui Wan with modifications. In cases with blood stasis, add *Radix Salviae Miltiorrhizae, Radix Paeoniae Rubra, Caulis Spatholobi* and *Herba Leonuri*; in cases with diverse bleeding, add *Herba Agrimoniae, Radix Rubiae, Colla Corii Asini, Herba seu Radix Cirsii* and *Herba Cephalanoploris*; in cases with fever, add *Rhizoma Coptidis, Radix Scultellariae, Cortex Phellodendri, Herba Taraxaci, Rhizoma Polygoni Cuspidati* and *Flos Lonicerae*.

Acupuncture treatment

1. For deficiency of *qi*, apply acupuncture and moxibustion to Xinshu (BL 15), Pishu (BL 20), Qihai (CV 6), Shenmen (HT 7) and Zusanli (S 36)

2. For deficiency of *yin*, apply acupuncture to Ganshu (BL 18), Shenshu (BL 23), Gaohuang (BL 43), Taixi (KI 3) and Sanyinjiao (SP 6).

3. For deficiency of *yang*, apply acupuncture and moxibustion to Dazhui (GV 14), Mingmen (GV 4), Shenshu (BL 23), Qihai (CV 6) and Zusanli (ST 36).

4. For bleeding, apply acupuncture to Geshu (B 17), Xuehai (SP 10), Yinbai (SP 1) and Chize (LU 5).

5. For diarrhea, apply acupuncture to Tianshu (ST 25).

6. For night sweating, apply acupuncture to Yinxi (HT 6).

7. For fever, apply acupuncture to Dazhui (GV 14) and Quchi (LI 11).

# MODERN RESEARCH

Over the past 30 years, researchers have studied 27 traditional Chinese prescriptions used to treat aplastic anemia. These prescriptions commonly contain the following ingredients: *Radix Codonopsis Pilosula, Radix Astragali, Rhizoma Atractylodis Macrocephalae*, Poria and *Radix Glycyrrhizae Praeparata* to strengthen *qi*; *Fructus Ligustri Lucidi, Fructus Lycii, Radix Polygoni Multiflori, Fructus Psoraleae, Cortex Cinnamomi, Plastrum Testudinis, Cortex Moutan Radicis* and *Rhizoma Rehmannia* to invigorate the kidneys; *Radix Angelicae Sinensis, Radix Paeoniae Alba* and *Caulis Spatholobi* to promote production of blood; and *Radix Codonopsis Pilosula* and *Radix Astragali* to replenish *yang* and promote hematopoiesis of red blood cells. In patients with seriously low red blood cell counts, add *Radix Ginseng, Radix Codonopsis Pilosula, Colla Corii Asini* and *Magnetitum*; in patients with leukopenia, add *Squama Manitis, Caulis Spatholobi, Rhizoma Polygoni Cuspidati, Fructus Psoraleae, Colla Cornus Cervi* and *Testa Arachidis*; for patients with thrombocytopenia, add *Folium Kaki, Herba Agrimo-*

*niae, Testa Arachidis* and *Fructus Forsythiae.*

Physicians at Xiyuan Hospital (Beijing) studied 169 cases of aplastic anemia treated with Decoction of Semen Cuscutae (composed of *Semen Cuscutae, Fructus Lycii, Fructus Corni, Fructus Ligustri Lucidi, Radix Polygoni Multiflori, Fructus Psoraleae, Herba Cistanchis, Fructus Mori, Radix Astragali* and *Radix Angelicae Sinensis*). The decoction achieved a practical cure in 23 (13.6 percent) of the 169 patients, remission in 57 (33.7 percent) and marked improvement in 61 (36.1 percent). Thus, the total effective rate was 83.4 percent (141 cases). Other studies showed that this prescription could remarkably raise the CFU-S, CFU-D and CFU-E levels in mice marrow inhibited by myleran, as well as increase the phagocytic rate and index of macrophage cells. This prescription can be given continuously for a long period without obvious side effects. This is important since aplastic anemia is a chronic disease and traditional Chinese medical treatment requires from six months to one year or more.

# CHAPTER XVII    LEUKEMIA

Acute leukemia is a primary malignant disease of the blood forming organs, characterized by a predominance of immature myeloid or lymphoid precursors (blasts). The blasts progressively replace the normal bone marrow, migrate, and invade other tissues. Production of normal erythrocytes, granulocytes and platelets diminishes, which leads to anemia, infection and hemorrhage.

Acute leukemia is classified morphologically according to the cell type involved: lymphocytic, myelocytic or monocytic. The mechanism of human leukemogenesis is unknown, but inciting agents are well established. These include ionizing radiation, oncogenic viruses, genetic and congenital factors and chemical agents. The clinical manifestations of acute leukemia relate to a decreased number of normal hematopoietic cells and invasion of other organs by leukemic cells. Anemia, hemorrhage, infection and leukemic infiltration are the most common pathologic changes.

Chronic leukemia shares the classifications of acute leukemia. The etiology of chronic leukemia is also unknown. In the early stages of the disease, patients are often asymptomatic, but their symptoms increase in the advanced stages. These include malaise, fatiguability, anorexia, weight loss, low-grade fever and night sweating.

## ETIOLOGY AND PATHOGENESIS

A weakened body resistance allows toxic heat to invade the body, which can lead to leukemia.

### 1. Internal injury of vital energy

Endogenous pathogenic factors may injure vital energy, leading to deficiency of *qi* and *yin*, manifested as anemia and hemorrhage.

### 2. Injury of blood by toxic heat

When the body's resistance is low, toxic heat may easily invade the body, impairing the bone marrow and blood and causing fever and heat syndromes.

## DIFFERENTIAL DIAGNOSIS OF SYNDROMES

### 1. Deficiency of *qi* and blood

Primary manifestations: Lassitude, pallor, shortness of breath, spontaneous sweating, headache, tinnitus, epistaxis, petechiae, ecchymoses, menorrhagia, pale tongue with thin, white coating and weak and rapid pulse; in some cases deficiency of both *qi* and *yin* may occur, manifested as lassitude, pallor, shortness of breath, spontaneous sweating, feverish sensation over the palms, soles and chest, reddened tongue with scanty coating and weak and rapid pulse.

**2. Injury of blood by toxic heat**

Primary manifestations: High fever, dry mouth and throat, preference for drinking, deep yellow urine, reddened tongue with yellowish and dry coating and floating and rapid pulse; in cases affected by damp heat, manifestations include fever, thirst without preference for drinking and reddened tongue with yellow, greasy coating.

## TREATMENT

**1. Deficiency of both *qi* and blood**

Principle of treatment: Invigorate *qi* and nourish blood.

Formula of choice: Bazhen Tang (Decoction of Eight Precious Ingredients) with modifications, including adding *Radix Ginseng*, R*adix Astrgali*, Poria and *Radix Glycyrrhizae* to invigorate *qi*; *Radix Angelicae Sinensis*, *Radix Paeoniae*, *Radix Rehmanniae* and *Colla Corii Asini* to nourish blood; and *Fructus Ligustri Lucidi* and *Semen Cuscutae* to replenish kidney *yin*. In cases with deficiency of *qi* and *yin*, add *Radix Scrophulariae, Radix Ophiopogonis, Herba Dendrobii* and *Cortex Moutan Radicis* to nourish *yin*.

**2. Injury of blood by toxic heat**

Principle of treatment: expel heat and detoxify.

Formula of choice: Qingwen Baidu Yin (Antipyretic and Antitoxic Decoction) with modifications; in cases with damp heat, add Haoqin Qingdan Tang (Sweet Wormwood and Scutellaria Decoction for Clearing Damp-Heat from the Gallbladder) with modifications; ingredients for this formula include: *Herba Artemisiae Chinghao, Indigo Naturalis, Radix Scutellariae, Rhizoma Coptidis* to remove damp-heat; *Rhizoma Pinelliae Praeparata*, Poria and *Radix Glycyrrhizae* to strengthen the spleen and eliminate damp; and *Fructus Aurantii* and *Pericarpium Citri Reticulatae* to regulate *qi* and eliminate dampness.

## MODERN RESEARCH

In one study, 259 patients with the acute non-lymphocytic leukemia received either Harringtonine (Har) or Homo-harringtonine (Hom) which had been extracted from *Cephalotaxus fortunei*. Complete remission among those who had received Har was 20 percent, and 22.3 percent among those who had received Hom. The effective rates were 72.7 and 63.8 percent, respectively. The complete remission rates of those who had received Har or Hom was higher than those of patients who had received 6-MP, MTX, CTX and drugs similar to Ara-C or DNR. Physicians at Suzhou Medical College observed the effect of Hom combined with VCR, Ara-C and prednisone (HOAP) on 278 cases of acute non-lymphocytic leukemia. The complete remission rate for this group was 60.1 percent, higher than that achieved with any other drugs.

Li, et al., reported on 110 patients with acute leukemia who received traditional medicine combined with chemotherapy. The prescription used consisted of *Radix Astragali, Radix Codonopsis Pilosula, Rhizoma Atractylodis Macrocephalae*, Poria, *Radix Rehmanniae, Radix Ophiopogonis, Radix Glycyrrhizae, Radix Asparagi, Rhizoma Polygoni Cuspidati, Herba Oldenlandiae Diffusae, Herba Scutellariae Barbatae, Herba Cephalanoploris* and *Cortex Moutan Radicis*. The therapy achieved a complete remission rate of 55.45 percent (61 cases), and a total effective rate of 76.4 percent (84 cases).

It should be noted that while increasing the effective rate of the therapy and dereasing the rate of relapse, the use of chemotherapy with traditional medicines also reduced chemotherapy's side effects.

Physicians have used indirubin, once isolated from *Indigo Naturalis* and now artificially synthesized, in treating chronic myelocyte leukemia. The Institute of Hematology under the Chinese Academy of Medical Sciences has observed 314 cases of chronic myelocoyte leukemia treated with indirubin. Physicians there found that the molecules of indirubin infiltrated into cytoplasm of leukemic cells to suppress the activity of DNA in the nucleus, thus leading to morphologic changes in the leukemic cells. Complete remission was observed in 82 cases (26.1 percent), partial remission in 105 cases (33.4 percent) and improvement in 87 cases (27.7 percent), for a total effective rate of 87.2 percent.

Zhou, et al., reported on 54 cases in which physicians used Qing Huang Powder, consisting of *Indigo Naturalis* and Realgar in proportions of either 9:1 or 7:3 to treat chronic myelocyte leukemia. The treatment achieved a remission rate of 70 percent (38 cases) and a partial remission of 28 percent (15 cases), for a total effective rate of 98 percent. Doctors found that Qing Huang inhibited the DNA and RNA synthesis of L615 and S180 cell strains. They discovered no side effects on periperal blood cells. Thus, the effective rate of indirubin and Qing Huang Powder in treating chronic myelocyte leukemia is similar to that of myleran but with fewer side effects.

# CHAPTER XVIII   IDIOPATHIC THROMBOCYTOPENIC PURPURA

Idiopathic thrombocytopenic purpura (ITP) includes acute and chronic immune thrombocytopenias in which there are no demonstrable underlying diseases. The main clinical features of ITP are the presence of petechiae and purpura, often accompanied by various types of bleeding, such as hemorrhagic bullae in the oral cavity and gastrointestinal and genitourinary bleeding. Traditional medical knowledge about "bleeding" can be applied to syndrome differentiation and treatment of ITP.

## ETIOLOGY AND PATHOGENESIS

### 1. Overabundance of epidemic heat
Overabundant epidemic heat may attack the body and invade the blood system, causing bleeding.

### 2. Interior heat due to *yin* deficiency
Edogenous heat caused by *yin* deficiency (known as interior heat) may invade the blood system, causing bleeding. *Yin* deficiency of the liver and kidneys is commonly seen.

### 3. Failure of *qi* to control blood
Under normal conditions, *qi* commands the blood circulating in the vessels. If *qi* is insufficient, it will fail to control the blood, resulting in bleeding.

## DIFFERENTIAL DIAGNOSIS OF SYNDROMES

### 1. Overabundance of epidemic heat
Primary manifestations: Petechiae and purpura caused by heat accumulated in the blood system usually occurring abruptly and accompanied by hemorrhagic bullae in the oral cavity, gastrointestinal and genitourinary bleeding, fever, dry mouth and thirst, deep yellow scanty urine, constipatioon, reddened tongue with yellow coating and rapid pulse. There is usually a history of an antecedent invasion by epidemic heat (upper respiratory infection) one-to-three weeks prior to the onset.

### 2. Interior heat due to *yin* deficiency
Primary manifestations: Disease begins insidiously with petechiae and purpura or other hemorrhages accompanied by feverish feeling in the palms, soles and chest, dry mouth, dizziness, ringing in the ears, irritability, insomnia, night sweating, reddened tongue with little or no coating and fine rapid pulse.

### 3. Failure of *qi* to control blood
Primary manifestations: Petechial hemorrhage and purpura accompanied by pallor,

lassitude, shortness of breath, spontaneous sweating, pale tongue with white coating and fine and weak pulse.

## TREATMENT

### 1. Overabundance of epidemic heat

Principle of treatment: Remove pathogenic heat and toxic materials from the body.

Formula of choice: Qingwen Baidu Yin (Antipyretic and Antitoxic Decoction) to expel heat and detoxify and cool the blood; in this formula, *Gypsum Fibrosum* and *Rhizoma Anemarrhenae* clear heat from the stomach; *Cornu Rhinoceri, Radix Rehmanniae, Radix Scrophulariae, Cortex Moutan Radicis* and *Radix Paeoniae Rubra* cool the blood and remove toxic materials; *Rhizoma Coptidis, Fructus Gardeniae* and *Radix Scutellariae* quench fire and detoxify; *Herba Lophatheri* removes fire from the heart.

### 2. Interior heat due to *yin* deficiency

Principle of treatment: Nourish *yin* and eliminate heat.

Formula of choice: Da Buyin Wan (Bolus for Replenishing Yin) in combination with Yiguan Jian (Ever-effective Decoction for Nourishing the Liver and Kidneys); in these two recipes, *Radix Rehmanniae, Plastrum Testudinis, Radix Ophiopogonis, Fructus Lycii* and *Radix Angelicae Sinensis* tonify the genuine *yin* of the liver and kidneys and soothe the liver; *Cortex Phellodendri* and *Rhizoma Anemarrhenae* eliminate pathogenic fire to protect *yin*; and *Fructus Meliae Toosenden* soothes the liver and regulates *qi*.

### 3. Failure of *qi* to control blood

Principle of treatment: replenish *qi* and guide blood to circulate within the vessels.

Formula of choice: Guipi Tang (Decoction for Invigorating the Spleen and Nourishing the Heart) with modifications; in this recipe, *Radix Ginseng, Radix Astragali, Rhizoma Atractylodis Macrocephalae*, Poria and *Radix Glycyrrhizae Praeparata* replenish *qi* and strengthen the spleen; *Radix Aucklandiae* regulates *qi*, enlivens the spleen and prevents the side effects of the drugs used to replenish *qi*; other ingredients in this recipe, such as *Arillus Longan* and *Semem Ziziphi Spinosis*, which nourish the heart and tranquilize the mind, may be subtrated when treating purpura.

Modifications: For cases with severe bleeding, add *Folium Artemisiae Argyi, Folium Biotae, Herba Agrimoniae*, and *Crinis Carbonisatus*; for cases with *yang* deficiency, add *Colla Cornus Cervi, Semen Cuscutae, Fructus Psoraleae* and *Rhizoma Curculiginis*.

## MODERN RESEARCH

Zheng Yisheng, et al., (Guiyang College of Traditional Chinese Medicine) reported on 80 cases of ITP treated with Decoction of *Fructus Gardeniae* and *Radix Rehmanniae*. The total effective rate in this study was 92.5 percent (76 cases). After treatment all patients got relief from hemorrhage, and their platelet counts increased to over one hundred thousand in 44 cases out of 80 (or 55 percent). The majority of patients received treatment for over three months.

Recently, Chinese physicians began to consider petechiae and ecchymosis signs of blood stasis, which has prompted them to focus on the role of drugs that promote blood circulaton and remove blood stasis in treating ITP. Their investigations have shown that drugs for removing blood stasis can inhibit anti-platelet antibody formation and immune reactions. Deng You'an, et al., (Chongqing Second People's Hospital) reported on 22 patients with ITP who received a prescription for removing blood stasis. The principal ingredients in this formula were *Radix Angelicae Sinensis, Rhizoma Ligustici Chuan-xiong, Radix Paeoniae Rubra, Flos Carthami, Caulis Spatholobi, Herba Leonuri, Radix Codonopsis Pilosulae* and *Radix Astragali*. Patients received one dose per day orally for seven to 66 days, for an average of 31 days. After treatment, five patients were markedly improved, and 15 patients showed some improvement, thus the total effective rate was 90.9 percent. Doctors performed a bone marrow examination in 15 cases before and after treatment and found that the production of blood platelet by mature megacaryocyte increased, the level of PA-IgG was reduced from $616.9 \pm 123.3$ pg/$10^7$ plat. to $213.6 \pm 113.3$ pg/$10^7$ plat. post-treatment. This study suggests that herbs for removing blood stasis have an immuno-suppressive effect, as well as the ability to regulate the balance between Th and Ts cells and strengthen the function of Ts cells. These drugs also reduced the fragility and permeability of capillaries. Since the pathogenesis of ITP is considered to be related to immune mechanisms, some physicians believe that therapy which removes blood stasis may be a key treatment for ITP.

Finally, Liu Tianji, et al., (Liaoning College of Traditional Chinese Medicine, Shenyang) studied 50 children with ITP. They treated Group 1 (15 cases) with herbal medicine based on differentiation of syndromes and Group 2 with herbal medicine and prednisone. The effective rate was 86.7 percent in Group 1 and 91.8 percent in Group 2. The combined therapy of traditional and Western medicines had little or no side effects and made it possible to shorten the course of treatment.

# CHAPTER XIX    DIABETES MELLITUS

Diabetes mellitus is a heterogeneous primary disorder affecting the processing of carbohydrates with multiple etiologic factors that generally involve absolute or relative insulin deficiency, insulin resistance or both. All causes of diabetes ultimately lead to hyperglycemia, which is the hallmark of this disease.

Diabetes is typically classified into Type I, or insulin dependent diabetes mellitus (IDDM), in which patients have little or no endogenous insulin secretory capacity, and Type II, or noninsulin-dependent diabetes mellitus (NIDDM), in which patients retain significant endogenous insulin secretory capacity.

Diabetes mellitus is known in traditional Chinese medicine as "Xiao Ke," a disease characterized by polydipsia, polyphagia and polyuria.

## ETIOLOGY AND PATHOGENESIS

Diabetes occurs in association with the following etiologic factors:

1. The spleen and stomach are damaged by overeating greasy food or by over-consuming alcohol, causing failure of the spleen in transporting and transforming which, in turn, causes interior-heat to accumulate and consume food and body fluids, finally resulting in diabetes.

2. Anxiety, anger and mental depression injure the liver, causing liver *qi* to stagnate. Protractedly stagnated liver *qi* turns into pathogenic heat which consumes body fluids and eventually leads to diabetes.

3. Deficiency in the kidneys caused by intemperance in sexual life or congenital essence defect causes kidney *qi* to wane; as a result, kidney *qi* fails to maintain the function of the bladder in restraining urine discharge, thus polyuria occurs.

## DIFFERENTIAL DIAGNOSIS OF SYNDROMES

Traditional Chinese medicine identifies three types of diabetes: upper, middle and lower. Differential diagnosis of syndromes is based on these three types.

**1. Diabetes involving the upper-*jiao***

Pathogenic heat consumes lung *yin*, thus affecting the upper-*jiao*.

Primary manifestations: Severe thirst accompanied by dryness of the mouth and tongue, polyuria, reddened tip and margin of the tongue with thin, yellow coating and full and rapid pulse.

**2. Diabetes involving the middle-*jiao***

Excessive fire of the stomach consumes stomach *yin*.

Primary manifestations: Polyphagia, emaciation, constipation, reddened tongue with dry, yellow coating and slippery and strong pulse.

### 3. Diabetes involving the lower-*jiao*

(1) *Yin* deficiency: A morbid state due to a defect in the kidney essence and consumption of kidney *yin*.

Primary manifestations: Polyuria, turbid urine, dry mouth, reddened tongue with little coating and weak and rapid pulse.

(2) Deficiency of both *yin* and *yang*: A morbid state due to deficiency of kidney *yin* and *yang*.

Primary manifestations: Severe polyuria, turbid urine, lassitude, spontaneous sweating, shortness of breath, impotence, dark complexion, pale tongue with white coating and sunken and weak pulse.

## TREATMENT

### 1. Diabetes involving the upper-*jiao*

Principle of treatment: Expel heat, purge fire, increase the production of body fluids and relieve thirst.

Formula of choice: Erdong Tang (Asparagus and Ophiopogon Decoction) with modifications; in this prescription, *Radix Asparagi* and *Radix Ophiopogonis* nourish *yin* of the lungs and stomach and promote the production of body fluids; *Radix Scutellariae* and *Rhizoma Anemarrhenae* clear away heat from the lungs and stomach; *Radix Ginseng* strengthens *qi* and produces body fluids; for patients with extreme thirst accompanied by a dry and yellow tongue coating, *Gypsum Fibrosum* can be prescribed to clear away stomach heat.

### 2. Diabetes involving the middle-*jiao*

Principle of treatment: Clear away stomach heat and nourish *yin*.

Formula of choice: Yunu Jian (Gypsum Decoction), in which *Gypsum Fibrosum* and *Rhizoma Anemarrhenae* clear away stomach heat; *Rhizoma Rehmanniae* and *Radix Ophiopogonis* nourish *yin* of the lungs and kidneys; and *Radix Achyranthis Bidentatae* brings fire downward; for cases with yellow, greasy tongue coating, add *Rhizoma Coptidis* and *Radix Scutellariae* to expel damp-heat from the stomach; for cases with constipation, add *Radix et Rhizoma Rhei, Cortex Magnoliae Officinalis* and *Fructus Aurantii Immaturus* to purge heat.

### 3. Diabetes involving the lower-*jiao*

(1) *Yin* deficiency:

Principle of treatment: Nourish kidney *yin*.

Formula of choice: Liuwei Dihuang Wan (Bolus of Six Ingredients Including Rehmannia); when this prescription is used to treat diabetes, use large dosages of *Fructus Corni, Radix Rehmanniae Praeparata* and *Rhizoma Dioscoreae* to nourish and retain *yin* of both the liver and kidneys and to replenish spleen *yin* in order to relieve polyuria.

(2) Deficiency of *qi* and *yin*:

Principle of treatment: Replenish *qi* and nourish *yin*.

Formula of choice: Liuwei Dihuang Wan (Bolus of Six Ingredients Including Rehmannia) and Shengmai San (Pulse-activating Powder); for patients with aversion to cold and cold limbs, add Shenqi Wan (Bolus for Tonifying Kidney *Qi*) to invigorate kidney *yin* and *yang*.

## MODERN RESEARCH

Kuang Ankun, et al., (Ruijin Hospital, Shanghai) observed the relationship between the levels of plasma estradiol ($E_2$), testosterone (T) and $E_2/T$ ratios and the differentiation of syndromes in traditional Chinese medicine. They found that $E_2$ and $E_2/T$ levels were higher and the T level was lower in male type II diabetics with *yang* or *yin* deficiency compared to normal male subjects. The authors assumed that an elevated $E_2/T$ level might represent a deficiency of the kidneys in male patients. They treated 22 cases of male type II diabetes with herbal drugs to replenish the kidneys for three months. (The basic prescription consisted of *Radix Codonopsis Pilosulae, Radix Astragali, Herba Epimedii, Semen Cuscutae, Fructus Lycii, Semen Biotae, Radix Rehmanniae, Stigma Maydis, Colla Prunus* and *Bombycis.*) After treatment, the elevated $E_2$ and $E_2/T$ levels tended towards normal and a remission of clinical symptoms occurred. The fasting blood glucose was reduced from 193.9±67.1mg/dl to 140.0±37.6 mg/dl.

Researchers of (Guang'anmen Hospital, Chinese Academy of Traditional Chinese Medicine, Beijing) observed the effects of Tablet A for Lowering Blood Glucose (TALBG) on diabetic. TALBG is composed of *Radix Astragali, Rhizoma Polygonati, Radix Rehmanniae* and *Radix Trichosanthis*. It is made into tablet form, with each tablet containing 2.3 g of the crude drug. Patients received six tablets orally three times a day. Doctors treated 405 cases of type II diabetes with TALBG for three months. They divided the patients into three groups: Group A (290 cases) suffered from deficiency of *qi* and *yin*, Group B (55 cases) from deficiency of *qi* and *yin* with excessive heat and Group C (60 cases) from deficiency of *yin* and *yang*. The effective rates were 81.4 percent, 65.6 percent and 63.3 percent and the fasting blood glucose decreased by 46.46±3.11, 40.71±6.55 and 44.69±7.29 mg/dl in Groups A, B and C, respectively. After ceasing the treatment, blood glucose levels elevated again. Doctors conducted a glucose tolerance test and determined the level of plasma insulin in 77 cases and found that the glucose tolerance improved and the level of plasma insulin increased significantly.

Ni Yanxia, et al., (No. 208 Hospital of the People's Liberation Army) demonstrated the effect of berberine on diabetes. They treated 60 cases of type II diabetes with 0.3-0.5 g berberine given orally once a day for one-to-three months. After treatment, the patients' fasting blood glucose levels were lowered from 208.65±51.68 mg/dl to 117.19±25.98 mg/dl.

Ni Yanxia and his associates carried out this study on rats with alloxon-induced diabetes. They divided the animals into Group A, the berberine group, and Group B, the control group. Group A received an intramuscular injection of 0.1 ml (2 mg) berberine once daily for 28 days. Group B received a similar dosage of normal saline. After 10 days' treatment, the average of blood glucose in Group B was 191.67 mg/dl and 98.35 mg/dl in Group A (P<0.01). Pathological examination of the rats' pancreases showed that the number of pancreas islands ß-cells in Group A was much larger than that of Groups B. The authors hypothesized that the hypoglycemic effect of berberine may be associated with its action in promoting regeneration and functional recovery of pancreas islands ß-cells.

Other research on the effects of traditional Chinese medicine found that *Radix Ginseng* not only reduced blood glucose but also adjusted the metabolism of blood lipid. In normal subjects, the level of plasma ß-lipoprotein was reduced and high density lipoprotein (HDL) was increased six hours after administering Ginseng powder. $Rb_2$, a Ginseng Saponin, decreased the level of plasma, total cholesterol and LDL.

Zu, et al., treated type-II diabetics with *Radix Salviae Miltiorrhizae* (36 g daily) for three months. The results indicated that its effect on anti-platelet aggregation was greater than that of dipyridamole (75-100 mg administered three times a day). Kong also found that in type-II diabetics, drugs that strengthen the kidneys can lower plasma $TXB_2$ level.

Chen reported that in patients with diabetes, increased blood viscosity could be decreased by acupuncture. The principal acupoints selected were Pishu (UB 20), Geshu (UB 17), Zusanli (ST 36), Feishu (UB 13), Weishu (UB 21) and Shenshu (UB 23).

While herbal medicines are most effective in treating patients with type-II diabetes, they may also be used with insulin to supplement the treatment of type-I diabetes, since herbal medicines may improve the patient's general condition.

# CHAPTER XX   HYPERTHYROIDISM
# (GRAVES' DISEASE)

Hyperthyroidism, or Graves' disease, is a morbid condition characterized by excessive quantities of circulating thyroid hormone that results in hypermetabolism. The precise etiology of Graves' disease is still unknown, but it is probably an auto-immune disorder in which an antibody stimulates human thyroid tissue. The stimulus for the antibody production remains obscure.

Graves' disease is marked by goiter, nervousness or tremors, weight loss (usually with increased appetite), palpitations, heat intolerance, excessive perspiration, emotional liability, muscle weakness and hyperdefecation.

## ETIOLOGY AND PATHOGENESIS

Traditional Chinese medicine considers emotional upset the cause of goiters. The mental state usually affects the functioning of *qi* and blood, which when disrupted can cause disorders of the visceral organs and lead to diseases. The following conditions are the common etiology of goiters.

1. Stagnated liver *qi* damages liver *yin*: Prolonged emotional depression can stagnate liver *qi*; protracted stagnation in turn leads to production of pathogenic heat, which causes excessive liver fire and which may attack *yin* of the stomach or the heart; deficiency of liver *qi* can lead to blood stasis, causing the thyroid gland to swell.

2. Liver fire attacks the stomach: Prolonged stagnation of liver *qi* may turn into liver fire. The stomach may be attacked by a transverse invasion of excessive liver fire, leading to deficiency of stomach *yin* due to *yin* overconsumption.

3. Anxiety impairs the heart: Since the heart controls mental and emotional activities, persistent anxiety will impair heart *yin*, leading to deficiency of heart *yin* and excessive heart fire.

In addition, deficiency of *qi* is often seen in advanced cases.

## DIFFERENTIAL DIAGNOSIS OF SYNDROMES

**1. Damage of liver *yin* by stagnated liver *qi***

Primary manifestations: Emotional depression or irritability, insomnia, distention in the hypochondriac region, a sensation of a foreign body in the throat, feverish sensation in the palms, soles and chest, reddened tongue with thin, white coating and small and rapid pulse.

**2. Deficiency of heart *yin* with excessive heart fire**

Primary manifestations: Restlessness, palpitations, insomnia, dream-disturbed sleep, amnesia, spontaneous sweating and/or night sweating, low fever, dry mouth, reddened tongue with little or no coating and thready and rapid pulse.

**3. Attack of the stomach by liver fire**

Primary manifestations: Irritability, flushed face, bitter taste in the mouth, dry throat, ringing in the ears, hungry feeling, constipation, weight loss, reddened tongue with yellow, greasy coating and slippery and rapid pulse.

**4. Deficiency of *qi* and *yin***

Primary manifestations: Lassitude, shortness of breath, weight loss and emaciation, loss of appetite, irritability, spontaneous and night sweating, slightly reddened tongue with thin, white coating and weak and rapid pulse.

## TREATMENT

**1. Damage of liver *yin* by stagnated liver *qi***

Principle of treatment: Regulate liver *qi* and nourish liver *yin*.

Formula of choice: Chaihu Shugan San (Bupleurum Powder for Relieving Liver *Qi*); this prescription, which regulates liver *qi* is used with *Radix Angelicae Sinensis* and *Radix Rehmanniae Praeparata* to nourish liver *yin*.

**2. Deficiency of heart *yin* with excessive heart fire**

Principle of treatment: Nourish *yin* and purge fire.

Formula of choice: Tianwang Buxin Dan (Cardiotonic Pill) and Niuhuang Qingxin Wan (Bezoar Sedative Bolus) with modifications; in these prescriptions, *Calculus Bovis* clears away heat from the heart; *Rhizoma Coptitis*, *Radix Scutellariae* and *Fructus Gardeniae* purge fire; *Radix Curcumae* regulates heart *qi*; *Semen Ziziphi Spinosae*, *Cinnabaris* and *Semen Biotae* induce tranquilization; *Radix Ophiopogonis*, *Radix Asparagi*, *Radix Scrophulariae* and *Fructus Schisandrae* nourish heart *yin*; and *Radix Angelicae Sinensis*, *Radix Rehmanniae* and *Radix Salviae Miltiorrhizae* replenish heart blood.

**3. Attack of the stomach by liver fire**

Principle of treatment: Purge liver fire and nourish stomach *yin*.

Formula of choice: Yiguan Jian (Ever-effective Decoction) with *Radix Bupleuri*, *Radix Scutellariae, Fructus Gardeniae* and *Radix Gentianae*; in this prescription *Radix Adenophorae Strictae* and *Fructus Lycii* replenish liver *yin*; and *Fructus Meliae Toosenden* regulates liver *qi* and expels liver heat.

**4. Deficiency of both *qi* and *yin***

Principle of treatment: Replenish *qi* and nourish *yin*.

Formula of choice: Buzhong Yiqi Tang (Decoction for Reinforing the Middle-*jiao* and Replenishing *Qi*) and Da Buyin Wan (Bolus for Replenishing *Yin*); in these prescriptions, *Radix Ginseng, Radix Astragali, Radix Atractylodis Macrocephalae* and *Radix Glycyrrhizae Praeparata* reinfore *qi* in the middle *jiao*; *Radix Rehmanniae Praeparata, Plastrum Testudinis* and the spinal marrow of pigs nourish liver and kidney *yin*; and *Cortex Phellodendri* and *Rhizoma Anemarrhenae* clear away fire from both the liver and kidneys.

Acupuncture treatment

Primary points: Jianshi (PC 5), Shenmen (HT 7), Sanyinjiao (SP 6), Taichong (LR

3), Taixi (KI 3), Fuliu (KI 7), Zusanli (ST 36), Neiguan (PC 6), Guanyuan (CV 4), Zhaohai (KI 6), Xinshu (BL 15), Ganshu (BL 18) and Shenshu (BL 23); these acupoints should be used according to the differentiation of syndromes; select three-to-four acupoints for each treatment.

## MODERN RESEARCH

According to modern clinical research, traditional Chinese medicine is indicated in the following conditions: mild and moderate hyperthyroidism; allergy to antithyroid drugs, such as derivatives of thiourea; hepatic diseases with complications; recurrences after discontinuance of antithyroid drugs; post-operative cases with poor response to antithyroid drugs; and progressive ophthalmopathy and enlarged thyroid despite use of antithyroid drugs.

Given that the majority of patients with hyperthyroidism have deficiency of *qi* and *yin*, doctors at Shanghai College of Traditional Chinese Medicine developed a prescription designed to replenish them consisting of *Radix Astragali* (45 g), *Spica Prunellae* (30 g), *Radix Paeoniae Alba*, *Radix Polygoni Multiflori* and *Radix Rehmanniae* (15 g each) and *Rhizoma Cyperi* (12 g). To this basic prescription, physicians added *Rhizoma Coptidis* for purging heart fire and *Radix Gentianae* for purging liver fire. In a comparative study of the basic prescription, doctors gave one group of patients the full formula and a second group the formula minus Astragalus. Both groups received one dose daily. The group which received the formula with Astragalus showed more improvement than the other group. Also, Astragalus improved the non-specific cellular immune function of the patients in the first group and their recurrence rate was lower than those in the second group, who did not receive Astragalus.

Yi Ningyu, et al., (Shanghai Second Medical University) demonstrated that the increased number of $\alpha$-adrenenergic receptors and the volume of oxygen consumption in an animal model of hyperthyroidism induced by $T_3$, could be normalized by administering *Radix Rehmanniae* and *Plastrum Testudinis*. These ingredients used with *Rhizoma Coptidis* to treat hyperthyroidism with *yin* deficiency and excessive heart fire provided symptomatic relief.

Kuang Ankun, et al., (Shanghai Second Medical University) explored the treatment of exophthalmus using the principle of replenishing *qi*, nourishing *yin* and clearing away heat from the liver. They used a prescription consisting of *Radix Ampelopsis*, *Radix Rhapontici seu Echinopsis*, *Radix Astragali*, *Herba Dendrobii*, *Flos Chrysanthemi*, *Fructus Lycii*, *Flos Buddlejae*, *Herba Senecionis Scandentis*, *Flos Eriocauli* and *Herba Dendrobii*. In some cases, they supplemented this formula with acupuncture or small dosages of tapazole and thyroxine. The prescription was effective 90.9 percent of the time in mild cases and 75 percent in moderate and severe cases. The degree of exophthalmus was reduced an average of 2.3 mm. Meanwhile, the levels of serum $T_3$ and $T_4$ were also lowered. The authors confirmed that the effectiveness of traditional Chinese medicine in treating exophthalmus is associated with its regulation of the immune and vegetative nervous functions.

Doctors have also studied the efficacy of acupuncture in treating hyperthyoidism.

Huo Jingseng, et al., (Shanghai College of Traditional Chinese Medicine) reported on 120 cases of hyperthyroidism. They treated 46 cases with acupuncture, 41 cases with tapazole (10 mg 4 times daily) and 33 cases with acupuncture and tapazole. The main acupoints was "*Qiyin*," a point located near Shuitu (ST 10), Neiguan (PC 6), Jianshi (PC 5), Zusanli (ST 36) and Sanyinjiao (SP 6). The acupuncture therapy was given once every other day for three months. The rates of clinical remission in the three groups were 47.8 percent, 65.9 percent and 81.8 percent, respectively. The relapse rates within one year were 36.4 percent, 88.9 percent and 29.6 percent, respectively, indicating that the combined therapy was most effective. Jing Shubai, et al., (Shanghai College of Traditional Chinese Medicine) also observed the effects of acupuncture on hyperthyroidism patients with exophthalmus. They treated 59 cases, including 108 eyes, with acupuncture, using Tianzhu (B 10) and Fengchi (B 20) as the main points, and Sanyinjiao (SP 6) and Taichong (LR 3) as supplementary points. Patients received acupuncture once every other day for three months. Of the 108 eyes treated, 37 (34.3 percent) recovered normal sight, 23 (21.3 percent) showed obvious improvement and 40 (37 percent) showed some improvement.

# CHAPTER XXI   CANCER

As elsewhere, cancer is one of the leading causes of death in China. It is characterized by the uncontrollable growth of cells originating from normal tissues which can kill the host by means of local extension or distant spread (metastasis). The etiology of cancer is not completely clear, but the fundamental mechanisms governing the etiology of human cancer have recently become clearer as new information about cancer genes, viruses, carcinogens, cell growth and differentiation emerges.

Over the past three decades, Chinese researchers have studied the role of traditional Chinese medicine in treating cancer. They have obtained significant results.

## ETIOLOGY AND PATHOGENESIS

### 1. Insufficient vital essence

Insufficient vital essence causes deficiency syndromes. Since various deficiency syndromes may occur in cancer patients, insufficient vital essence is considered the basic pathogenesis of cancers. Insufficient vital essence results from congenital defects, senility, protracted illness, overexertion, improper diet, over indulgence in sexual activity or invasion by exogenous pathogenic factors.

### 2. Blood stasis and phlegm accumulation

Traditional Chinese medicine holds that cancerous tumours are the result of blood stasis or phlegm accumulation or both. *Qi* activates and governs blood circulation. Deficiency of *qi* may cause blood stasis. Stagnation of *qi*, which is usually due to an emotional upset or affection by exopathogens, is another common factor that impedes the normal flow of blood and results in blood stasis and eventually tumour formation. Accumulation of phlegm is related to the various deficiency states described above, particularly deficiency of spleen *qi* characterized by failure in transporting and transforming the refined substances from food and water which leads to the formation of phlegm.

### 3. Invasion of exogenous pathogenic factors

Exogenous pathogenic heat or cold can invade the body, disturb the smooth flow of *qi* and blood and, as a result, cause the retention of *qi* and blood and the formation of tumours.

## DIFFERENTIAL DIAGNOSIS OF SYNDROMES

### 1. *Qi* deficiency

Primary manifestations: General lassitude, shortness of breath, laboured breathing and speaking, spontaneous sweating that worsens on exertion, pale tongue with thin, white coating and weak pulse.

Conditions associated with cough and expectoration of copious thin sputum indicate a deficiency of lung *qi*; poor appetite, fullness in the abdomen after meals, loose stools or edema indicate a deficiency of spleen *qi*; palpitations or arrhythmia may appear in cases with deficiency of heart *qi*.

### 2. *Yang* deficiency

Primary manifestations: Intolerance of cold, cold limbs, slow pulse with the manifestations of *qi* deficiency.

Deficiency of kidney *yang* is manifested as weakness of the loins and knees, impotence, frequent urination at night, incontinence of urine, diarrhea before dawn or edema complicated by the general manifestations of *yang* deficiency.

### 3. Blood deficiency

Primary manifestations: Pallor or sallow complexion, pale tongue with thin, white coating and thready pulse. Additional manifestations may include palpitations, insomnia, amnesia and dream-disturbed sleep, suggesting deficiency of heart blood; blurred vision, dizziness, ringing in the ears, numbness of the hands and feet or scanty menstrual flow, indicate deficiency of liver blood.

### 4. *Yin* deficiency

Primary manifestations: Dry mouth with preference for beverages, absence of tongue coating, constipation and concentrated urine, indicating consumption of body fluids; feverish sensation in the palms, soles and chest, afternoon fever, night sweating, deep red tongue without coating and fine rapid pulse, suggesting interior heat due to *yin* deficiency. Patients with *yin* deficiency, suffering from restlessness, dizziness, dryness of the eyes, nocturnal emissions, sourness and weakness of the loins and knees, can be diagnosed as having *yin* deficiency of the liver and kidneys. Those with *yin* deficiency, suffering from dry cough or cough with expectoration of scanty, sticky sputum, can be diagnosed as having *yin* deficiency of the lungs.

### 5. Stagnation of liver *qi*

Primary manifestations: Fullness and distending pain in the hypochondriac regions, irritability, belching, loss of appetite, distending sensation in the breast, thin, white tongue coating and taut pulse.

### 6. Blood stasis

Primary manifestations: Fixed pain or mass in a given region of the body, petechiae or bleeding, dark complexion, dry scaly skin, dysmenorrhea with discharge of dark-red blood or clots, purple or dark-red tongue and fine and hesitant pulse.

### 7. Phlegm-dampness

Primary manifestations: Cough, expectoration of mucoid white sputum, loss of appetite, abdominal distention, white, greasy tongue coating and slippery pulse.

## TREATMENT

### 1. *Qi* deficiency

Principle of treatment: Invigorate *qi*.

Formula of choice: Si Junzi Tang (Decoction of Four Noble Drugs). The most commonly used herbs to tonify *qi*: *Radix Ginseng*, *Radix Codonopsis Pilosulae* and *Radix*

*Astragali*. For deficiency of lung *qi*, use Bufei Tang (Lung-Tonifying Decoction), in which *Radix Ginseng* and *Radix Astragali* replenish lung *qi*, *Cortex Mori Radicis* and *Radix Asteris* descend lung *qi* and *Radix Rehmanniae Praeparata* and *Fructus Schisandrae* invigorate the kidneys, the root of *qi*.

For deficiency of spleen *qi*, Shen Ling Baizhu San (Powder of Ginseng, Poria and White Atractylodes) is an effective formula. It includes the ingredients of the Decoction of Four Noble Drugs, as well as *Semen Delichoris Album*, *Rhizoma Dioscoreae*, *Semen Coicis* and *Semen Nelumbinis* which invigorate spleen *qi*; *Fructus Amomi* which enlivens the spleen and strengthens the action of the principal drugs; and *Radix Platycodi* which acts as a guiding drug. For the cases with deficiency of heart *qi*, use Yangxin Tang (Decoction for Nourishing the Heart), in which *Radix Ginseng*, *Radix Astragali*, *Radix Glycyrrhizae* and *Fructus Schisandrae* replenish heart *qi*; *Cortex Cinnamomi* invigorates heart *yang*; *Radix Angelicae Sinensis* and *Rhizoma Ligustici Chuanxiong* nourish heart blood; and *Semen Ziziphi Spinosae*, Poria, *Radix Polygalae* and *Semen Biotae* ease the mind.

## 2. *Yang* deficiency

Principle of treatment: Replenish *yang* with herbs warm in nature.

Formula of choice: Fuzi Lizhong Tang (Decoction for Regulating Middle-*jiao* with Aconite) for deficiency of spleen *yang*; in this formula, *Radix Aconiti* and *Rhizoma Zingiberis Praeparata*, both of which are pungent in flavour and hot in property, restore *yang* of the spleen and stomach by warming the middle-*jiao* to dispel cold; add *Radix Ginseng*, *Radix Atractylodis Macrocephalae* and *Radix Glycyrrhizae* to replenish *qi* and strengthen the spleen.

Yougui Yin (Kidney-Yang Reinforcing Decoction) is an effective recipe for treating deficiency of kidney *yang*.

## 3. Blood deficiency

Principle of treatment: Nourish blood.

Formula of choice: Siwu Tang (Decoction of Four Ingredients) to replenish liver blood; the treatment of blood deficiency is usually combined with herbs that invigorate *qi* and nourish the kidneys, for example, Danggui Buxue Tang (Chinese Angelica Decoction for Replenishing Blood), which includes a large dosage of *Radix Astragali*; Guipi Tang (Decoction for Invigorating the Spleen and Nourishing the Heart) is frequently prescribed for deficiency of heart blood.

## 4. *Yin* deficiency

Principle of of treatment: Nourish *yin* and increase body fluids.

Formula of choice: Since *yin* deficiency frequently causes heat, methods for nourishing *yin* are often used with those for expelling heat; use Da Bu Yuan Jian (Potent Decoction for Replenishing Orignial Essence) to treat *yin* deficiency of the liver and kidneys, in which *Radix Ginseng*, *Rhizoma Disocoreae* and *Radix Glycyrrhizae* replenish the spleen, *Radix Rehmanniae Praeparata* and *Radix Angelicae Sinensis* nourish liver *yin* and *Fructus Corni* and *Fructus Lycii* invigorate kidney *yin*.

Deficiency of lung *yin* can be treated with Baihe Gujin Tang (Lily Decoction for Strengthening the Lungs), in which *Radix Rehmanniae* nourishes *yin* and clears away heat from the blood; *Radix Ophiopogonis, Radix Scrophulariae* and *Bulbus Licii* nourish *yin*, moisten the lungs, remove phlegm and arrest cough; *Radix Angelicae Sinensis* and *Radix Paeoniae Alba* invigorate blood and nourish *yin*; and *Radix Glycyrrhizae* and *Radix Platycodi* eliminate phlegm and coordinate the effects of the other ingredients in the formula.

### 5. Stagnation of liver *qi*

Principle of treatment: Regulate liver *qi*.

Formula of choice: Chaihu Shugan San (Bupleurum Powder for Soothing Liver *Qi*).

### 6. Blood stasis

Principle of treatment: Promote blood circulation to remove blood stasis.

Formula of choice: Gexia Zhuyu Tang (Decoction for Dissipating Blood Stasis Under the Diaphragm), in which *Radix Angelicae Sinensis, Rhizoma Ligustici Chuanxiong, Radix Paeoniae Rubra, Semen Persicae, Flos Carthami, Faeces Trogopterorum* and *Cortex Moutan Radicis* promote blood circulation to remove blood stasis, and *Rhizoma Cyperi, Fructus Aurantii, Radix Linderae* and *Rhizoma Corydalis* regulate *qi* to alleviate pain.

### 7. Phlegm-dampness

Principle of treatment: Remove dampness and phlegm.

Formula of choice: Pingwei San (Peptic Powder) and Liu Junzi Tang (Decoction of Six Noble Ingredients); in these recipes, *Radix Ginseng, Radix Atractylodis*, Poria and *Radix Glycyrrhizae* invigorate *qi*, strengthen the spleen and eliminate dampness; *Exocarpium Citri Grandis*, and *Rhizoma Pinelliae* are added to remove dampness, *Cortex Magnoliae Officinalis* and *Pericarpium Citri Reticulatae* to regulate *qi* and dispel wetness and *Rhizoma Zingiberis Recens* and *Ziziphi Jujubae* to regulate the function of the stomach.

## MODERN RESEARCH

Sun Yan, et al., (Cancer Institute, the Chinese Academy of Medical Sciences, Beijing) demonstrated that traditional Chinese medicine could help some cancer patients live longer.

They employed two recipes, both for strengthening body resistance. One is composed of *Radix Astragali* (30 g), *Fructus Ligustri Lucidi, Radix Angelicae Sinensis, Caulis Spatholobi, Fructus Lycii* (15 g each) and *Pericarpium Citri Reticulatae* (6 g). Physicians extracted these ingredients and made them into tablets, 0.5 g for each tablet (equivalent to 3 g of the crude drug), and administered 8-10 tablets three times a day orally daily. The other contains *Radix Astragali* (30 g) and *Rhizoma Polygonati, Caulis Spatholobi, Semen Cusculae* and *Fructus Ligustri Lucidis* (15 g each). It was prepared and administrated in the same way as the first recipe. Through ten-year follow-up thrity-two of the 43 patients with carcinoma of the uterine cervix or the breast who received radiation combined with herbal recipe survived, whereas only 23 of 46 patients who received radiation alone survived.

Zhou Agao, et al., (Shanghai Second Medical University) observed the efficacy of the Modified Small Golden Pill combined with chemotherapy in treating patients in the intermediate and late stages of gastric cancer after they had been operated on. Doctors randomly divided 72 cases into a therapeutic group and a control group. The two groups were similar in sex and age composition and clinical manifestations and surgical operations received. One month after their operations, patients in both groups received the same chemotherapy except that the control group did not take Modified Small Golden Pills.

Modified Small Golden Pills consist of *Semen Strycyni* (0.5 g), *Radix Angelicae Sinensis, Resina Commiphorae Myrrhae* (6g each), *Lumbricus, Faeces Trogopterorum, Radix Salviae Miltiorrhizae, Radix Aconiti Kusnezoffii Praeparata, Pericarpium Citri Reticulatae, Cortex Magnoliae Officinalis, Radix Aucklandiae* (9 g each). Doctors made these ingredients into tablets, 0.4 g each tablet, and gave them orally in a dosage of four tablets, three times a day. The patients in both groups received FT-207 (100-200 mg) three times a day. The survival rate after one, one-and-a-half and two years was 93.2 percent, 82.4 percent and 80.0 percent, respectively, in the therapeutic group, and 64.3 percent, 48.0 percent and 38.9 percent, respectively, in the control group.

Qiu Jiaxin, et al., (Longhua Hospital, Shanghai) observed the efficacy of the therapeutic method in strengthening the spleen, regulating *qi*, eliminating heat and phlegm and softening hard lumps in the late stages of liver cancer. Physcians primarily used *Radix Codonopsis Pilosulae* or *Radix Pseudostellariae, Rhizoma Atractylodis Macrocephalae Praeparata*, Poria, *Cortex Moutan Radicis, Flos Lonicerae, Radix Kalimeridis, Concha Ostreae, Spica Prunellae, Squama Manitis Praeparata, Carapax Trionycis, Flos Rosae Rugosae, Lumbricus* and *Rhizoma Arisaematis* prepared in a decoction given orally once a day. They treated 129 cases with this recipe as the therapeutic group and 97 cases with other therapy as the control group. The survival rate for one year in patients with primary liver cancer was 31 percent in the therapeutic group and 4.5 percent in the control group, $P < 0.05$; in the cases of secondary cancer of the liver, the survival rate was 33.8 percent in the therapeutic group and 16 percent in the control group, $P < 0.05$. Doctors also used a mutation assay (V79 cell) for the initiation model and metabolic cooperation for the promotion model to determine whether the multi-stage concept of carcinogenesis (initiation and promotion) could be influenced by these herbal medicines. The results showed that some Chinese medical herbs do have anti-mutation and anti-promotion effects, as well as cytotoxicity on human liver cancer cells (7402).

Chen Liming, et al., (Fuzhou Institute of Medical Sciences) reported on 49 cases of primary liver cancer treated with AT2, an extract of cockroach. Another 46 cases received traditional Chinese medicine combined with Western medicine as the control group. Among the AT2 group, symptoms (including hepatic pain, anorexia, emaciation, abdominal distension and lassitude) were relieved, hepatomegaly was reduced, AFP levels were lowered and the life spans of these patients were prolonged. The half-year and one-year survival rates for the AT2 group were 31.91 percent and 14.89 percent, respectivly and 8.7 percent and 0 percent, respectively, in the control group. The AT2 group also experienced no toxic side effects on the heart, liver, or kidneys; the only side effect some patients experienced was dryness in the mouth.

Further experimental studies indicated that the inhibitory effect of AT2 on tumour growth in S180 and S37 mice were 44-52 percent and 34.05-42.1 percent, respectively. In the cells of S180 and ESC mice, the inhibitory effects of tumour growth were 50-60 percent and 30-55 percent, respectively. The macrophage phagocytosis of the peritoneal cavity of mice was also enhanced and the weight of the spleen increased.

Ning Chunhong, et al., (Guang'anmen Hospital, Chinese Academy of Traditional Chinese Medicine, Beijing) reported on their approach to relieving the toxic reactions of postoperative chemotherapy in patients with advanced gastric carcinoma. They studied 326 cases of gastric carcinoma diagnosed pathologically as stage III to IV without metastasis to other internal organs. One hundred eighty cases received traditional Chinese medicine and chemotherapy as the therapeutic group, 146 cases received only chemotherapy as the control group.

Both groups were treated by the FMV programme (5-Fluorouracil, Mitomycin and Vincritin) for four-to-six weeks. Since the principle of treatment in this case is to strengthen the spleen and replenish the kidneys, the doctors used *Radix Codonopsis Pilosulae, Radix Atractylodis Macrocephalae, Fructus Psoraleae, Fructus Ligustri Lucidi* and *Fructus Lycii*.

The five year survival rate for stage III gastric carcinoma patients was 51.7 percent in the therapeutic group and 31.2 percent in the control group. In the therapeutic group, 95 percent of the patients completed their chemotherapy course with fewer side effects than patients in the control group experienced. The combined therapy also improved the patients' immuno-function.

Pao Menji, et al., (Fuzhou Red Cross Society Hospital) reported on 150 cases of nesopharyngeal carcinoma treated with a combination of traditional Chinese medicine and radiation. The prescription used consisted of *Radix Ophiopogonis, Radix Adenophorae Strictae, Radix Angelicae Sinensis,* Poria, *Rhizoma Atractylodis Macrocephalae, Radix Glycyrrhizae, Radix Asparagi, Rhizoma Imperatae, Radix Codonopsis Pilosulae, Radix Scrophulariae, Rhizoma Polygonati Odorati, Flos Lonicerae, Herba Oldenlandiae Diffusae* and *Radix Salviae Miltiorrhizae,* prepared in a decoction. The survival rate after three years among these patients was 72 percent 58 percent after five years and 30.8 percent after 10 years.

The Cancer Hospital of the Chinese Academy of Medical Sciences compared the efficacy of traditional Chinese medicine and radiation in treating nasopharyngeal cancer to that of radiation only. Doctors treated 92 patients with the combined therapy and 105 patients with radiation only as the control group. They used *Radix Astragali, Radix Paeoniae Rubra, Rhizoma Ligustici Chuanxiong, Semen Persicae, Flos Carthami, Radix Puerariae, Radix Angelicae Sinensis, Caulis Spatholobi, Radix Salviae Miltiorrhizae* and *Pericarpium Citri Reticulatae,* prepared in decoction. Survival rates for one, three, and five years later were 91.3 percent, 67.4 percent and 52.5 percent, respectively, in the combined treatment group, and 80 percent, 33.3 percent and 24 percent, respectively, in the control group.

In summary, traditional Chinese medicine has proven to be an effective tool for treating cancer. It can strengthen the patient's body resistance and raise the immuno-function, inhibit cancer formation or metastasis, increase the efficacy of chemotherapy and radiation, reduce the side effects of chemotherapy and radiation, and prolong survival time.

Chinese physicians have also focused their research on the mechanisms of traditional Chinese medicine which make it effective in treating cancer. Hu, et al., found that *Radix Codonopsis Pilosulae* given alone did not inhibit the growth of subcutaneously transplanted Lewis lung tumour and its metastatic foci in Swiss mice, but when used with a small dose of Cyclophosphamidum (20 mg/kg), it became effective. Specifically, the median survival time became longer, $33.24 \pm 1.31$ days in the *Codonopsis Pilosula* group compared to $28.0 \pm 1.35$ days in the control group. Also, the tumours in the first group became smaller and their spontaneous metastatic foci fewer.

Wei, et al., investigated the effect of the Decoction for Invigorating Body Resistance and Expelling Toxic Materials on the tumour necrosis factor produced by peritoneal macrophages of normal and EMT6 solid tumour-bearing mice. Cyclophosphamidum and lipopolysaccharide were used as the controls. The results showed that in vitro, lipopolysaccharide could induce tumour necrosis factor production. Medicinal herbs and cyclophosphamidum were unable to induce tumour necrosis factor production, but if these were given in combination, the production of tumour necrosis factor by the peritoneal macrophages of tumour-bearing mice increased.

The medicinal herbs used in this experiement were *Radix Astragali, Radix Rehmanniae, Radix Ophiopogonis, Pericarpium Citri Reticulatae, Flos Lonicerae, Caulis Bambusae in Taeniam, Rhizoma Atractylodis Macrocephalae* and *Fructus Ligustri Lucidi*. Other studies have shown that some herbal medicines for promoting blood stasis, such as *Rhizoma Zedoariae, Rhizoma Sparganii, Radix Angelicae Sinensis, Rhizoma Ligustici Chuanxiong, Flos Carthami, Radix Paeoniae Rubra, Eupolyphaga seu Steleophaga, Hirudo* and *Squama Manitis* can inhibit the growth of tumours to some extent.

Lu, et al., observed the anti-cancer biological effect of Naphthoqinone Pigment-LIII, a single substance extracted from *Arnebia Euchroma*. They found that Naphthoquinone Pigment-LIII could inhibit the proliferation of the stomach cancer cell line and the esophagus cancer cell line. At the effective concentration of 5 μg/ml, the mitotic index and growth curve declined without showing any damage to normal cells. At 5-10 μg/ml, the colony efficiency of cancer cells became significantly lower. Researchers believe the anti-cancer effect of Naphthoquinone Pigment-LIII may be related to its role in influencing the amount of RNA and the ultrastructure of cancer cells.

Zhu, et al., reported on the effects of berbamine on tumours in mice. Berbamine is an alkaloid extracted from *Berberis Poiretii Schn.* After the doctors hypodermically transplanted S180 cells and intraperitoneally transplanted HAC and EAC ascitic tumour cells into three different groups of mice, they gave the mice in the berbamine group 20 mg/kg berbamine intraperitoneally, once daily for ten days. As a result, the growth inhibitory rate was 75-78 percent in the mice with the S180 tumour cells, and the life-span extension rate was 68-80 percent in the HAC and EAC groups. Light and electron microscopic examination showed that there were necrosis and metabolic disturbances in the tumour cells treated by berbamine. The $LD_{50}$ of berbamine was $112 \pm 0.04$ mg/kg by peritoneal injection.

Hu, et al., have studied the anticarcinogenic activation of α-Asarone on human carcinoma cells. α-Asarone (C12H1603) is refined from the volatile oil of *Acorus Calamus*. The results showed that α-Asarone could kill human cancer cells, including SGC-7901 (gastric cancer cells), Detroit-6 (esophageal cancer cells) and Hela (cervix uteri cancer cells). The effective dosage of α-Asarone on $ED_{50}$ of SGC cells was about 25 μg/ml. α-Asarone caused a series of morphological changes in human carcinoma cells which both damaged them and inhibited their multiplication.

Researchers have also studied the preventive effects of traditional Chinese medicine on cancer. Jiang, et al., investigated the efficacy of Liuwei Dihuang Wan (Bolus of Six Ingredients Containing Rehmannia) in preventing cancer of the esophagus. They observed 507 patients with severe esophageal epithelial, all of whom lived in a region with a high incidence of esophageal carcinoma. They divided these patients randomly into two groups: Groups A (290 cases) received the herbal medicine at a dose of two boluses, twice daily for two years; Group B (217 cases) received no medicine. Through 10-year follow-ups, the incidence of esophageal carcinoma was 1.4 percent in Group A, and 7 percent in Group B.

Jiang, et al., also followed 1,097 cases of chronic hepatitis with positive AFP. They treated 270 of these patients with traditional Chinese medicine. After one year, the incidence of liver cancer was 2.6 percent among those who had received the herbal treatment and 8.5 percent among those who had not.

Over the past 30 years, doctors have screened more than 3,000 herbs and 200 recipes for their anti-cancer effects. The results of these examinations indicated that some herbal medicines can directly kill cancer cells. They are: *Rabdosia Rubescens* and *Rubescensine A and B*; *Brucea Javanica* and its oil or emulsion preparation; *Sophora Alopecuroides*; *Sophocarpine*; *Marsdenia Tenaccissima*; *Aconitum Carmichaeli* and *Acontine*; *Mylabris Phalerata* and the derivatives of *Cantharidin* and *Disodium Cantharidinate*; *Lycoris Radiate*; *Lycorine*; *Sarcandra Glaber* and its flavone; *Cephalotaxus Fortunei*; and Harringtonine.

# CHAPTER XXII    ARTERIAL HYPERTENSION

Systemic arterial hypertension is defined as elevated arterial blood pressure, with systolic pressure over 160 mmHg and/or diastolic pressure over 95 mmHg. Blood pressure that is consistently 140 mmHg systolic and/or 90 mmHg diastolic or higher is considered border line hypertension.

Hypertension is usually of two types: primary and secondary. Essential, or primary, hypertension is systemic arterial hypertension of unknown cause; 90 to 95 percent of systemic hypertension cases fall under this category. Seconary hypertension is elevated systemic blood pressure of known cause; five to 10 percent of systemic hypertension cases are of this type. In this chapter, we discuss only the traditional diagnosis and treatment of essential hypertension.

In traditional Chinese medicine, essential hypertension is included in the syndromes of headache and dizziness due to interior injury.

## ETIOLOGY AND PATHOGENESIS

### 1. Hyperactivity of liver-*yang*
The liver is related to mental activities, such as thinking and worrying. Mental upset or a fit of anger may cause hyperactivity of liver *yang*, and as a result, headache or dizziness occurs. On the other hand, excessive liver *yang* may turn into fire, which in turn, injures liver *yin* and eventually leads to hyperactivity of liver *yang*.

### 2. Deficiency of both *qi* and blood
Under normal conditions, *qi* and blood nourish the brain. Overstrain and stress may damage the function of the heart and spleen. As a result, *qi* and blood production is insufficient, which fails to nourish the brain and gives rise to headaches or dizziness.

### 3. Deficiency in the kidneys
The kidneys use their essence to produce marrow, and the brain is the sea of marrow. Deficiency in the kidneys impairs their ability to produce enough marrow to nourish the brain, thus dizziness or headaches may occur.

### 4. Interior retention of phlegm-damp
Improper diet, overwork and stress or a protracted illness may impair the spleen and stomach in transporting and transforming, which results in the production of damp and phlegm. Stagnant phlegm-damp, impeding the ascending of pure *qi* and the desending of turbid *yin*, causes dizziness or headaches.

## DIFFERENTIAL DIAGNOSIS OF SYNDROMES

### 1. Hyperactivity of liver *yang*
Primary manifestations: Headache or dizziness aggravated by mental upset, irritabil-

ity, flushed face, tinnitus, dry mouth with bitter taste, dream-disturbed sleep, reddened tongue with yellow coating and taut, rapid pulse.

### 2. Deficiency of *qi* and blood

Primary manifestations: Headache or dizziness with lassitude, shortness of breath, palpitations, insomnia, spontaneous sweating, pink tongue with thin, white coating and taut and thready pulse. (This morbid condition usually occurs in patients with hypertension complicated by cardiac dysfunction).

### 3. Deficiency in the kidneys

Primary manifestations: Headache or dizziness accompanied by an empty feeling of the head, tinnitus, weakness of the lower back and knees, impotence or nocturnal emissions, dry mouth, reddened tongue with little coating and fine and weak pulse.

### 4. Interior retention of phlegm-damp

Primary manifestations: Headache or dizziness with a heavy and tight feeling in the head, a feeling of fullness and oppression over the chest and epigastrium, loss of appetite, somnolence, corpulent tongue with white, greasy coating and soft and slippery pulse.

## TREATMENT

### 1. Hyperactivity of live *yang*

Principle of treatment: Calm the liver and suppress exuberant *yang*.

Formula of choice: Tianma Gouteng Yin (Decoction of Gastrodia and Uncaria) with modifications; in this recipe, *Rhizoma Gastrodiae*, *Rhizoma Uncariae cum Uncis*, *Concha Haliotidis* and Poria (Prepared with Cinnabar) calm the liver and suppress exuberant *yang*; *Fructus Gardeniae* and *Radix Scutellariae* clear away heat from the liver and strengthen the effect of calming the liver; and *Radix Cyathulae*, *Cortex Eucommiae* and *Ramulus Loranthi* nourish the kidneys to regulate the liver. In cases with flushed face, bloodshot eyes, bitter taste in the mouth, dry throat, yellow, greasy tongue coating and signs of a flaring-up of liver fire, use Longdan Xiegan Tang (Decoction of Gentiana for Purging Liver Fire).

### 2. Deficiency of *qi* and blood

Principle of treatment: Replenish *qi* and nourish blood.

Formula of choice: Bu Zhong Yi Qi Tang (Decoction for Reinforcing Middle-*jiao* and Replenishing *Qi*) plus *Herba Asari*, *Fructus Viticis* and *Rhizoma Ligustici Chuanxiong* for replenishing *qi* and expelling wind in patients suffering mainly from *qi* deficiency; Siwu Tang (Decoction of Four Ingredients) puls *Flos Chrysanthemi* and *Fructus Viticis* should be used with patients with headaches due predominantly to blood deficiency to nourish blood and eliminate wind.

### 3. Deficiency in the kidneys

Principle of treatment: Invigorate the kidneys.

Formula of choice: Qi Ju Dihuang Wan (Bolus of Rehmannia with Wolfberry and Chrysanthemum); this prescription is composed of Liuwei Dihuang Wan (Bolus of Six Drugs Including Rehmannia), which nourishes kidney *yin*, and *Fructus Lycii* (Wolfberry) and *Flos Chrysanthemi*, which nourish and calm the the liver; for patients with deficiency of kidney *yang*, use Yougui Wan (Kidney-*yang* Reinforcing Bolus), while for patients with deficiency of kidney *yin*, use Zuogui Wan (Kidney-*yin* Replenishing Bolus).

**4. Interior retention of phlegm-damp**

Principle of treatment: Eliminate damp and dissolve phlegm.

Formula of choice: Banxia Baizhu Tianma Tang (Decoction of Pinellia, White Atractylodes and Gastrodia), in which *Pericarpium Citri Reticulatae*, *Rhizoma Pinelliae*, Poria and *Radix Glycyrrhizae* dissolve phlegm; *Rhizoma Gastrodiae* and *Fructus Viticis* calm the liver and expel wind; *Rhizoma Atractylodis Macrocephalae* and *Fructus Ziziphi Jujubae* regulate the middle-*jiao* and strengthen the spleen to enforce the effect of dissolving phlegm-damp.

Acupuncture treatment

1. Points used to calm liver *yang* are: Fengchi (GB 20), Baihui (GV 20), Xuanlu (GB 5), Xiaxi (GB 43) and Xingjian (LR 2), manipulated with the reducing method.

2. Points to replenish and regulate *qi* and blood are: Baihui (GV 20), Qihai (CV 6), Ganshu (BL 18), Pishu (BL 20), Shenshu (BL 23) and Zusanli (ST 36), manipulated with the reinforcing method.

3. Points to tonify the kidneys are: Baihui (GV 20), Shenshu (BL 23), Sanyinjiao (SP 6), Fengchi (GB 20), Qihai (CV 6), Taixi (KI 3) and Guanyuan (CV 4), manipulated with the reinforcing method.

4. Points to resolve phlegm and eliminate damp are: Baihui (GV 20), Fengchi (GB 20), Touwei (ST 8), Pishu (BL 20), Zhongwan (CV 12), Neiguan (PC 6) and Fenglong (ST 40), manipulated with the reducing method.

# MODERN RESEARCH

Most traditional physicians believe that the principal pathogenesis of hypertension is a disturbance between *yin* and *yang*. The common syndrome types are hyperactivity of *yang* due to *yin* deficiency, hyperactivity of liver fire and deficiency of *yin* and *yang*. Hypertension is closely related to disorders of the liver, kidneys and heart. Research has shown that treatment of hypertension based on differentiation of syndromes is effective in about 90 percent of cases, especially in improving clinical symptoms, such as headache, dizziness and tinnitus.

Physicians of Shanghai Shuguang Hospital treated 832 cases of primary hypertension with Decoction of Curculigo and Epimedium. Eighty percent of the cases achieved a stable efficacy of antihypertension, relief from symptoms and no side effects. The decoction is composed of *Radix Curculiginis*, *Herba Epimedii*. *Radix Morindae Officinalis*, *Cotex Phellodendri*, *Radix Angelicae Sinensis* and *Rhizoma Anemarrhenae*, and is especially indicated for female hypertensive patients with climacteric manifestations.

Recent researches have found the following herbs or their extracts have an antihypertensive effect.

Tetrandrine, an effective alkaloid extracted from *Radix Stephaniae Tetrandrae*, can be given intravenously for severe hypertension or malignant hypertension at a dose of 120-180 mg. It can also be administered orally in long-term treatment of primary hypertension at a dose of 100 mg, three times a day. Studies have shown its effective rate to be 69 percent, yet it does not cause postural hypotension or other side effects, or impair the liver and kidneys.

*Folium Apocyni Veneti* is also an effective herb for hypertension. It is usually taken as a drink in a dose of 3-6 g per day. In one study of dogs with perinephritic hypertension, their blood pressure was lowered from 194/142 mmHg to 152/100 mmHg two hours after oral administration of *Folium Apocyni Veneti*, and it remained at a lower level for three days. No severe side effects were found, but weakness and dizziness occurred in some cases.

While *Ramulus Uncariae cum Uncis* is a medicinal herbal often administered to calm the liver and clear away heat, clinical and experimental studies have also demonstrated its anti-hypertensive effect. The component in *Ramulus Uncariae cum Uncis* which reduces blood pressure is Rhynchophylline. It is indicated for treatment of mild and moderate hypertension.

*Radix Aristolochiae* has a hypotensive action, its main component for lowering blood pressure being Magnoflorine. It has an obvious ganglion-blocking effect but without special selectivity. Thus, it is not a satisfactory substitute for other ganglionic antagonists.

Results from experimental studies in animal models of hypertension showed that the following traditional Chinese medicines have anti-hypertensive action: *Radix Puerariae, Flos Chrysanthemi Indici, Lumbricus, Rhizoma Coptidis, Radix Scutellariae, Cortex Phellodendri, Cortex Eucommiae, Cortex Moutan Radicis, Rhizoma Corydalis Decumbentis* and *Radix Adenophorae Strictae*.

*Qigong* (breathing exercise) therapy has also shown promise in relieving hypertension. Kuang Ankun, et al., randomly divided 204 patients with essential hypertension into two groups: 104 cases received *Qigong* therapy plus a small amount of hypotensor and 100 cases in the control group received a small amount of Western hypotensor only. Two months after treatment the hypotensive effect rate was 91 percent both in the *Qigong* group and in the contol group. One year later, it was 92 percent in the *Qigong* group and 80 percent in the control group. Twenty years later it was 88 percent in the *Qigong* group and 67 percent in the control group. During the 20 years doctors followed the progess of these patients, they found that the incidence of stroke and the rate of mortality were 16.35 percent and 11.54 percent, respectively, in the *Qigong* group, and 30 percent and 23 percent, respectively, in the control group. These studies showed that *Qigong* played a major role in improving the self-regulation function and in relieving multiple cerebro-cardiovascular risk factors.

In general, traditional treatment of hypertension lowers the blood pressure less but relieves hypertensive symptoms better than Western medicines. Therefore, combined traditional Chinese medicine and Western medicine is a logical approach for hypertension.

# CHAPTER XXIII   VIRAL MYOCARDITIS

Viral myocarditis is frequently caused by Group B coxsackie viruses, and less often by Group A coxsackie viruses.

Myocarditis often goes unrecognized, either because of its subclinical nature or because of the severity of associated conditions. The only clinical manifestation may be electrocardiographic change. Less commonly, cardiac enlargement and decreased exercise tolerance may occur. If symptomatic, the patient may complain of fever, palpitations, pleuropericardial pain, dyspnea, edema or fatigue. Or, the patient may die suddenly.

## ETIOLOGY AND PATHOGENESIS

According to traditional medical theory, viral myocarditis is caused by an attack of epidemic heat, which invades the body through the pores, skin, mouth and nose, and enters the lungs, and finally the heart, resulting in impaired heart *qi* or heart *yang*, or consumption of *yin*.

## DIFFERENTIAL DIAGNOSIS OF SYNDROMES

### 1. Retention of epidemic heat in the heart

Occurs in the acute stage of myocarditis, after an upper respiratory infection.

Primary manifestations: Low fever, spontaneous sweating, palpitations, constipation, deep yellow urine, reddened tongue with yellow coating and rapid pulse often associated with arrhythmia.

### 2. Deficiency of heart *qi*

Primary manifestations: Lassitude, pale complexion, palpitations, shortness of breath, pale tongue with thin coating and fine, weak pulse often complicated by arrhythmia.

### 3. Deficiency of heart *qi* and *yin*

Primary manifestations: Lassitude, shortness of breath, palpitations, feverish sensation in the palms and soles, dry mouth, reddened tongue with little coating and fine and rapid pulse frequently associated with arrhythmia.

### 4. *Yang* deficiency of the heart and kidneys

Primary manifestations: Lassitude, shortness of breath, palpitations, pale complexion, intolerance to cold, cold limbs, pale tongue with white coating and fine, weak pulse with arrhythmia or slow pulse.

## TREATMENT

### 1. Retention of epidemic heat in the heart

Principle of treatment: Clear away the epidemic heat from the heart.

Formula of choice: Qing Wen Bai Du Yin (Antipyretic and Antitoxic Decoction); in this prescription, *Radix Rehmanniae*, *Rhizoma Coptidis*, *Radix Paeoniae Rubra*, *Fructus Forsythiae*, *Radix Scrophulariae*, *Cortex Moutan Radicis* and *Herba Lophatheri* cool blood and clear away heat from the heart; other ingredients clear away pyretic factors. (*Cornu Rhinoceri* may be omitted because of its high price.)

**2. Deficiency of heart *qi***

Principle of treatment: Replenish heart *qi*.

Formula of choice: Danggui Buxue Tang (Chinese Angelica Decoction for Replenishing Blood), in which *Radix Astragali* replenishes heart *qi* and *Radix Angelicae Sinensis* nourishes the heart blood; if the patients are susceptible to cold, use Jade-Screen Powder; in this prescription, *Radix Astragali* invigorates *qi* and strengthens the body's superfical resistance; *Rhizoma Atractylodis Macrocephalae* strengthens the spleen and increases *qi* and blood and *Radix Ledebouriellae* and *Radix Astragali* increase the action of strengthening the superfical portion of the body.

**3. Deficiency of heart *qi* and *yin***

Principle of treatment: Replenish *qi* and nourish *yin*.

Formula of choice: Shengmai San (Pulse-activating Powder); in this recipe, *Radix Ginseng* replenishes heart *qi*; and *Radix Ophiopogonis* and *Fructus Schisandrae* nourish heart *yin*.

**4. *Yang* deficiency of the heart and kidneys**

Principle of treatment: Warm and invigorate the heart and kidneys.

Formula of choice: Qi Fu Tang (Astragalus and Aconite Decoction); in this recipe *Radix Astragali* invigorates the heart *qi* and Radix Aconiti warms the kidney *yang*.

# MODERN RESEARCH

Chen Shuxia, et al., (Shanghai Second Medical University) observed the therapeutic effect of Yupingfeng San (Jade-screen Powder) and Shengmai Ye (Pulse-activating Solution) on Coxsackie B viral myocarditis. They gave 30 patients Jade-screen Powder (15 g twice a day orally) and Pulse-activating Solution (10 ml twice a day orally) for two to three months; another 20 normal volunteers received Jade-screen Powder (15g twice a day orally for one week) as the control group.

After the treatment, clincial symptoms were relieved. Abnormal changes in the ECG, such as sinus tachycardia, frequent ventricular premature heart beat, paroxysms of ventricular tachycardia and sino-artrial block, also improved dramatically.

Doctors determined the activity of natural killer (NK) cells before and after treatment. Before treatment, the NK activity in 24 cases (80 percent) was lower than that of the normal subjects. After treatment with traditional Chinese medicine, NK activity was elevated from $12.26\pm1.31$ percent to $31.99\pm4.23$ percent.

Yang Yinzhen, et al., (Zhongshan Hospital, Shanghai Medical University) reported on a controlled study of the efficacy of Astragalus in treating Coxsackie B viral myocarditis. One group of patients received Astragalus granules (16.5 g twice a day orally for three months), while another group received conventional Western therapy (polarized liquid, coenzyme A, vitamin C, etc.). Improvement of the left ventricular function was greater in the Astragalus group than in the control group.

Another series of patients with Coxsackie B viral myocarditis received Astragalus injections intrasmuscularly in a dosage of 4ml (derived from 8 g of crude Astragalus root) daily for three to four months. NK cell activity, depressed before treatment, was remarkably increased at the end of the treatment, while in the conventional therapy group no such improvement was observed. The therapeutic nature of Astragalus was also shown by its effect on the electric activity of Coxsackie B-2 virus-infected rat myocardial cells in culture, as the occurrence of premature beats, tachycardia and fibrillation was much rarer in the myocardial cells treated with Astragalus.

Rong Yizhi, et al., (Sanhua Hospital, Shanghai Medical University) reported that Pulse-activating Powder can protect the myocardium from damage caused by adriamycin (an anti-cancer drug). Gong, et al., observed the protective effect of ginsenoside on the beating myocardial cell cultures of neonatal rats. Cultured under the conditions of insufficient glucose and hypoxia, the myocardial cells treated with ginsenoside had much better histologic findings, ultrastructures and activity of succinate dehydrogenase than those of the control group.

# CHAPTER XXIV   CORONARY HEART DISEASE

Coronary heart disease (CHD), also known as ischemic heart disease, is commonly caused by atheromatous lesions of the coronary artery. Its major clinical manifestations are angina pectoris and myocardial infarction.

Although the terms angina pectoris and acute myocardial infarction were not used in ancient times, descriptions of the clinical manifestations of coronary heart disease are contained in the ancient texts of traditional Chinese medicine.

## ETIOLOGY AND PATHOGENESIS

Precordial pain is the most prominent feature of coronary heart disease. According to traditional medical theory, obstruction in the heart vessels usually causes this pain. The vessels may be blocked by phlegm accumulated in the chest, which obstructs *yang-qi*, and/or by blood stasis either due to *qi* deficiency or due to *qi* stagnation.

## DIFFERENTIAL DIAGNOSIS OF SYNDROMES

### 1. Obstruction of *yang-qi* in the chest due to accumulation of phlegm

Primary manifestations: A feeling of oppression over the chest or chest pain radiating to the back, accompanied by shortness of breath, white, thick, greasy coating of the tongue and smooth pulse. (This condition is of the cold phlegm type; when the tongue coating turns yellow and greasy, it becomes a phlegm-heat type.)

### 2. Blood stasis caused by *qi* deficiency

Primary manifestations: Fatigue, shortness of breath, palpitations accompanied by localized pain, dark purplish tongue with thin coating and uneven pulse. (In cases with cold extremities, intolerance of cold, pale and tender tongue and slow pulse, the blood stasis is due to *yang* deficiency; in cases with profuse sweating, deadly cold limbs, listlessness and fading pulse or even coma, the *yang* is exhausted and shock ensues. Some patients experience *yin* and *qi* deficiencies together, manifested by a heat sensation in the palms and soles, dry mouth, desire for cold drink, reddened tongue with little or no coating and thin, rapid pulse.)

### 3. Blood stasis caused by *qi* stagnation

Primary manifestations: A fullness sensation or pain in the chest, dark purplish tongue with thin coating, but no symptoms of *qi* deficeincy, such as shortness of breath and fatigue.

## TREATMENT

### 1. Obstruction of *yang-qi* in the chest due to accumulation of phlegm

Principle of treatment: Relieve the obstruction of *yang-qi* in the chest.

Formula of choice: Gualou Xiebai Baijiu Tang (Decoction of Trichosanthes and Allium with Wine); in this prescription, *Fructus Trichosanthis* eliminates phlegm and reverses the adverse ascending of *qi*; *Bulbus Allii Macrostemi* warms and activates *yang-qi* in the chest and relieves pain; and the wine acts as a guide drug.

### 2. Blood stasis caused by *qi* deficiency

Principle of treatment: Invigorate *qi* and promote blood circulation.

Formula of choice: Buyang Huanwu Tang (Decoction Invigorating *Yang* for Recuperation); in this recipe, *Radix Astragali* invigorates *qi* to promote blood circulation and strengthens the effect of the other ingredients in removing blood stasis.

In cases with *yang* deficiency, add *Semen Cuscutae, Radix Aconiti Praeparata*, and *Fructus Psoraleae* to warm and replenish *yang-qi*.

If there is collapse, use Shen Fu Tang (Decoction of Ginseng and Aconite) and Fuzi Tang (Aconite Decoction); in these prescriptions, *Radix Aconiti Lateralis Praeparata* and *Radix Ginseng* recuperate depleted *yang* and replenish *qi*.

In cases of *qi* and *yin* deficiencies add *Radix Scrophulariae, Radix Ophiopogonis, Fructus Schisandrae* and *Radix Rehmanniae* to the above prescriptions.

### 3. Blood stasis caused by *qi* stagnation

Principle of treatment: Activate *qi* and remove blood stasis.

Formula of choice: Xuefu Zhuyu Tang (Decoction for Dissipating Blood Stasis in the Chest); in this recipe, *Fructus Aurantii* and *Radix Bupleuri* activate stagnated *qi*; *Radix Platycodi* acts as a guide drug; and the other ingredients promote blood circulation and remove blood stasis.

Acupuncture treatment

Primary acupoints: Tanzhong (CV 17), Juque (CV 14), Neiguan (PC 6) and Xinshu (BL 15).

Supplementary acupoints:

For *qi* stagnation: Add Qimen (LR 14) and Taichong (LR 3).

For phlegm accumulation: Add Zusanli (ST 36) and Fenglong (ST 40) to strengthen the function of the spleen and resolve phlegm.

For *yang* deficiency: Add Shenshu (BL 23) and Taixi (KI 3) with the reinforcing method to warm kidney *yang* and invigorate kidney *qi*.

For *yin* deficiency: Add Sanyinjiao (SP 6) to adjust the *qi* of the three *yin* meridians.

## MODERN RESEARCH

Since 1970, doctors have conducted a number of studies on the use of traditional Chinese medicine in treating coronary heart disease (CHD). These investigations determined the beneficial effects of many Chinese herbal drugs, leading to their wide use in treating CHD in China. The most commonly used therapeutic principles, recipes and drugs are listed below.

### 1. The principle for replenishing *qi* and activating blood flow

As *qi* deficiency and blood stasis are the most common syndrome patterns in CHD, the therapeutic principle of replenishing *qi* and activating blood is frequently applied. The drugs used for this purpose are:

(1) Injection for *Qi* and Blood (IQB), composed of *Radix Ginseng, Radix Astragali* and *Radix Angelica Sinensis*. Its clinical efficacy was observed by a placebo-controlled single-blind crossover trial. The total effective rate of IQB for angina pectoris was 90.6 percent, while in the placebo group, the effective rate was only 16.6 percent. Improvement of ischemic ST-T changes was found in 56.25 percent of the IQB group and 11.1 percent of the placebo group. The submaximal treadmill exercise test further showed the efficacy of IQB. The exercise duration in the IQB group increased from 348.50 to 503.5 M, but remained unchanged in the placebo group.

(2) Anti-Myocardial Infarction Mixture (AMIM), a prescription for replenishing *qi* and promoting blood flow which consists of six herbal drugs: *Radix Astragali, Radix Codonopsis Pilosulae, Rhizoma Polygonati, Radix Salviae Miltiorrhizae, Radix Paeoniae Rubra* and *Radix Curcumae*. Doctors randomly divided 430 patients with acute myocardial infarction (AMI) into two groups. Group A (215 cases) received AMIM in combination with Western drugs; Group B received Western drugs alone. The mortality during hospitalization was 6.5 percent in Group A and 14.9 percent in Group B. Further analysis revealed that AMIM therapy reduced the mortality rate due to shock and heart failure.

### 2. The principle for promoting blood circulation to remove blood stasis

Physicians tested a mixture called "Coronary Heart No. II" (CH-II), consisting of *Radix Salviae Miltiorrhizae, Rhizoma Ligustici Chuanxiong, Radix Paeoniae Rubra, Flos Carthami* and *Lignum Dalbergiae Oderiferae*, on 112 patients with angina pectoris using a placebo-controlled double-blind crossover trial. The frequency and severity of angina attacks decreased in 80 percent of the patients in the CH-II group, and the dosage of nitroglycerine required was significantly reduced in 44.2 percent of the patients, while in the placebo group these changes occurred in 16.1 percent and 20.5 percent of the patients, respectively.

Compound Salivia Miltiorrhiza Injection is a simplified preparation derived from CH-II, containing only *Radix Salviae Miltiorrhizae* and *Lignum Dalbergiae Oderiferae*. It is indicated in cases of frequent and severe angina episodes and acute myocardial infarction, because it can be administered intravenously and takes effect rapidly. After use of this injection, angina episodes greatly improved in 62.1 percent of the patients, as did ischemic ECG in 50.9 percent of the patients. No side effects were recorded.

Doctors have isolated a few of the active substances for promoting blood circulation from the drugs, such as Tanshinone II-A sodium sulfonate (TS-IIA), Danshensu, Danshen diterpenes (DS-781), 3,4-Dihydroxyacetophenone and Sodium ferulate. Some chemical synthetics (e.g., Tetramethylpyrazine) are now available for clinical use.

### 3. The principle for replenishing *qi* and nourishing *yin*

The representative formula is Shengmai San (Pulse-activating Powder), consisting of *Radix Ginseng, Radix Ophiopogonis* and *Fructus Schisandrae*. It is indicated for patients with deficiency of *qi* and *yin*.

### 4. The principle for replenishing *qi* and warming *yang*

This principle is applied to CHD patients with deficiency of *qi* and *yang*. The preparation used is called Heart-strengthening Decoction, which consists of *Radix Aconiti*

*Lateralis Praeparata* and *Radix Astragali* as the chief ingredients.

**5. The principle for removing blood stasis with drugs warm in nature and aromatic in flavour**

The preparations in this category provide rapid relief of angina attacks and are often used in acute episodes. Aromatics warm in nature, such as *Resina Liguidambaris Orientalis, Lignum Santali* and *Benzoinum*, promptly activate the flow of *qi* to remove blood stasis and relieve pain. Liquidambar Coronary Pill, Moschus Heart Pill, Heart-pain Aerosol and *Kuan Xiong* Aerosol are examples of this type of preparation. They take effect within three to five minutes, which is comparable to nitroglycerin, but have no side effects.

In summary, while the therapeutic mechanisms of traditional Chinese medicines used to treat CHD may have different pharmacologic actions, their common actions are: (1) to lower blood viscosity and increase the myocardial nutrient blood flow; (2) to increase the plasma 6-keto-$PGF_1\alpha$ level; (3) to inhibit the adhesion and aggregation of platelets and decrease the plasma $TXB_2$, ß-TG, $PF_4$ level; (4) to strengthen left ventricular performance; and (5) to increase 2,3-DPG level in the hemoglobin.

# CHAPTER XXV    HEART FAILURE

Heart failure is a pathophysiologic state in which the left and/or right ventricles fail to pump adequate quantities of blood needed to meet the metabolic requirements of the various organs of the body, especially during stress or exercise. A wide spectrum of diseases, such as rheumatic heart disease, coronary heart disease, arterial hypertension and cardiomyopathies, can result in heart failure.

Heart failure is generally identified by its duration (acute or chronic), initiating mechanisms and the ventricle that is primarily affected. The most common clinical categories of heart failure are as follows:

### 1. Acute or chronic heart failure

Heart failure usually begins insidiously, but in some patients it occurs abruptly, such as after acute myocardial infarction, and is thus called acute heart failure.

### 2. Left or right heart failure

In heart failure one ventricle always fails before the other. In coronary heart disease and arterial hypertension, heart failure usually begins with the left ventricle. On the contrary, in rheumatic mitral stenosis, heart failure usually begins with the right ventricle.

The symptoms of heart failure are related to the ventricle involved and the duration of the failure. Left ventricular failure is characterized by pulmonary congestion and edema, right ventricular failure by systemic venous congestion and peripheral edema.

## ETIOLOGY AND PATHOGENESIS

### 1. Attack of exogenous pathogenic factors

Exogenous pathogenic factors may invade the superficies of the body and accumulate in the meridians and attack the blood system, which disturbs blood circulation and causes cardiac dysfunction.

### 2. *Qi* deficiency of the heart and spleen due to overstrain or anxiety

If overstrain or anxiety injures the heart and spleen, these viscera will become deficient in *qi*.

*Qi* is the dynamic force behind blood circulation. When *qi* is insufficient, blood circulation is impaired, resulting in blood stasis.

### 3. *Yang* deficiency of the spleen and kidneys

If *qi* deficiency of the heart and spleen persists for a long time, it further deteriorates and causes *yang* deficiency, especially of the spleen and kidneys.

When spleen *yang* is insufficient, the spleen fails to transport and transform food and fluids. As a result, accumulation of water leads to edema. The pathogenic water affects the heart and causes palpitations. The accumulated water also attacks the lungs, leading to cough, expectoration of sputum, shortness of breath and dyspnea.

# DIFFERENTIAL DIAGNOSIS OF SYNDROMES

### 1. Deficiency of heart *qi* (an early syndrome of heart failure)

Primary manifestations: Lassitude, shortness of breath, spontaneous sweating, palpitations that worsen upon exertion, pale tongue with teeth marks on its margin, thin, white tongue coating and weak pulse or arrhythmia.

### 2. Deficiency of both *qi* and *yin*

Primary manifestations: Lassitude, shortness of breath, palpitations, reddened tongue with little or no coating, dry mouth, preference for beverages, feverish sensation in the palms and soles and fine rapid pulse or arrhythmia.

### 3. Blood stasis due to *qi* deficiency

Primary manifestations: Gloomy complexion, palpitations, shortness of breath, lassitude, stabbing pain in the chest, dilation of neck veins, mass in the upper abdomen, thin, white tongue coating, dark purple lips and tongue sometimes marked by ecchymoses and uneven pulse or arrhythmia.

### 4. Retention of fluid due to *yang* deficiency

Primary manifestations: Palpitations, shortness of breath or dyspnea, cough with expectoration of sputum, edema, lassitude, intolerance of cold, cold limbs, swollen pale tongue with white coating and deep or slow pulse.

# TREATMENT

### 1. Deficiency of heart *qi*

Principle of treatment: Replenish heart *qi*.

Formula of choice: Buzhong Yiqi Tang (Decoction for Reinforcing Middle-*jiao* and Replenishing *Qi*), in which *Radix Ginseng*, *Radix Astragali*, *Radix Glycyrrhizae* and *Rhizoma Atractylodis Macrocephalae* replenish heart *qi*; *Radix Angelicae Sinensis* nourishes heart blood; and *Rhizoma Cimicifugae* and *Radix Bupleuri* raise the pure *qi* and strengthen the effect of tonifying *qi*.

### 2. Deficiency of both qi and *yin*

Principle of treatment: Replenish *qi* and nourish *yin*.

Formula of choice: Shengmai San (Pulse-activating Powder).

### 3. BLood stasis due to *qi* deficiency

Principle of treatment: Replenish *qi* and promote blood circulation to remove stasis.

Formula of chocie: Buyang Huanwu Tang (Decoction for Invigorating *Yang* and Recuperation); in this recipe, Astragalus, the principal herb, is usually given in a dose of 30g or more; the other ingredients promote blood circulation to remove blood stasis; Astragalus also helps diuresis; *Herba Leonuri* and *Herba Lycopi* remove blood stasis and promote diuresis and may be used if there is edema.

### 4. Retention of water-damp due to *yang* deficiency

Principle of treatment: Warm *yang* and promote diuresis, i.e. remove excessive body fluids through urination by invigorating the spleen and kidney *yang* with herbal drugs of warm property.

Formula of choice: Guizhi Fuzi Tang (Decoction of Cinnamon Twig and Aconite) and Wuling San (Powder of Five Drugs with Poria) with modifications; in these prescriptions, *Ramulus Cinnamomi*, *Radix Aconiti Praeparata* and *Rhizoma Zingiberis* warm *yang*; Poria, *Polyporus Umbellatus*, *Rhizoma Atractylodis Macrocephalae*, *Rhizoma Alismatis* and *Radix Glycyrrhizae* replenish the spleen to induce diuresis.

# MODERN RESEARCH

Since the founding of the People's Republic of China, physicians have studied the inotropic effects of herbs upon the heart. They have found more than 30 kinds of traditional herbal drugs that contain a variety of cardiac glucosides which increase myocardial contractions.

Research conducted on several of these herbs is described below.

### 1. Decoction of Codonopsis, Astragalus and Strophanthus

Yi Waijue, et al., (Dongzhimen Hospital, Beijing College of Traditional Chinese Medicine) used this prescription to treat chronic heart failure. It is composed of *Radix Astragali*, *Radix Codonopsis Pilosulae*, *Herba Lycopi*, *Herba Leonuri*, *Strophanthus Divaricatus*, Poria, *Rhizoma Zingiberis Recens* and *Rhizoma Pinelliae*. In this prescription, *Radix Codonopsis Pilosulae* and *Radix Astragali* replenish *qi*, *Herba Lycopi* and *Herba Leonuri* promote blood circulation, and the other ingredients are used in the diuretic formula Wupi Yin (Decoction of Five Drugs).

These doctors used this decoction to treat 33 patients with congestive heart failure (mostly of classes III and IV, as formulated by the New York Heart Association) caused by rheumatic heart disease or coronary heart disease. Patients received only this recipe once per day and no other cardiotonic drugs, such as digitalis. Thirty-one patients got relief from clinical manifestations of heart failure, such as dyspnea, palpitations, cough with expectoration of sputum and edema, within an average of five days. This decoction also significantly decreased auricular fibrillation in patients whose ventricular rate was rapid and refractory to digitalis therapy. Doctors also found that the 4-6 g of *Strophanthus Divaricatus* used in this recipe contains a Strophanthin-like glycoside which is better at blocking atrioventricular conduction than digoxin is. Gastrointestinal disorders, which occurred in four cases, and second degree atrioventricular block, which occurred in two cases, were the most common adverse reactions to *Straphanthus Divaricatus* and were quickly reversible after dose reduction or discontinuance of the herb.

### 2. Sheng Mai San

Sheng Mai San (Pulse-activating Powder) is a famous prescription for replenishing *qi* and nourishing *yin*. Liao Jiazhen, et al., (Dongzhimen Hospita, Beijing) reported on its effect on left ventricular performance in coronary heart disease (CHD) observed by means of systolic and diastolic time intervals (STI and DTI, also termed mechanocardiogram). The diagnosis of CHD was made according to the criteria formulated by the World Health Organization.

Doctors divided 76 cases of CHD randomly into three groups. Group A's 54 patients received 10 ml of Sheng Mai San (SMS), containing Ginseng (1 g), *Radix Ophiopogonis* (0.31 g), *Fructus Schisandrae* (0.15 g) mixed with 10ml of 10 percent dextrose, intravenously. Group B's 10 patients received 0.6 mg of cedilanid-D mixed with 10ml of 10 percent dextrose, given intravenously as the control group of the positive inotropic drug. Group C's 12 patients received only 20 ml of 10 percent dextrose intravenously as the placebo control group. An additional 30 normal subjects served as the normal control. Doctors recorded mechanocardiograms one hour before and one hour after administering medications and the placebo. SMS exerted a positive inotropic effect on the heart as reflected in improved systolic and diastolic time intervals. These effects are summarized as follows:

(1) Heart rate: The heart rate after SMS administration was slower, while the blood pressure showed no significant change, which suggests that SMS reduced the myocardial oxygen consumption.

(2) PEP/LVET ratio: The PEP/LVET ratio is inversely correlated with cardiac stroke. During heart failure, an increase in the PEP/LVET ratio occurred; after SMS administration, the PEP/LVET ratio decreased significantly, indicating an improvement of left ventricular performance.

(3) a/H percent ratio and LVEDP (left ventricular end diastolic pressure): The a/H percent ratio is an important index of the left ventricular compliance. After SMS administration the a/H percent ratio in Group A diminished, particularly in patients with hypertension, indicating an improvement in left ventricular compliance and a decrease in LVEDP.

In addition, Liao Jiazhen, et al., treated 22 cases of acute myocardial infarction admitted within 48 hours after onset of the condition with 10 ml SMS intravenously. The PEP/LVET ratio in these patients was reduced from $0.54\pm0.04$ (pre-treatment) to $0.48\pm0.02$ (post-treatment).

Doctors also carried out a placebo-controlled single-blind crossover trial on 14 patients with heart failure to observe the effect of SMS on the heart using a computerized nuclear stethoscope. Patients in the control group received a 20 ml 5 percent glucose solution intravenously as the placebo. One hour before and one hour after administering either glucose solution or SMS, doctors measured the left ventricular function.

The results showed that SMS increased the ejection fraction (EF), the relative cardiac output (RCO) and the stroke volume (SV). The effects started at 10 minutes and peaked at 20 minutes after administering the medication. The EF value increased from $0.35\pm0.02$ to $0.42\pm0.02$ 30 minutes after administering SMS. Doctors observed no changes in the placebo group.

Other studies on the mechanisms of SMS responsible for positive inotropic effect have yielded the following results.

(1) The activity of $(Na^+ - K^+)$ ATPase was inhibited by $24.98\pm5.23$ percent at a dose of 0.3 ml of SMS in vitro.

(2) The plasma cAMP level decreased from $41.92\pm6.22$ Pmole/ml to $28.31\pm4.7$ Pmole/ml in patients with acute myocardial infarction. As Krause noted, after acute myocardial ischemia, the first biochemical response is an increase in plasma level of cAMP, which may be related to the increased adrenergic activity. The ability of SMS to reduce high cAMP levels in plasma suggests the improvement of acute myocardic

ischemia or a decrease in the adrenergic activity.

(3) The effect of SMS on 2,3-diphosphoglyceric acid (2,3-DPG) levels in hemoglobin was studied in normal subjects and rats in vivo. In normal subjects, 24 hours after intravenous injection of 10 ml SMS, the 2,3-DPG level in hemoglobin increased from $14.15\pm0.44$ to $16.29\pm0.5$ ($\mu M/g$). In the rats that received SMS at a dose of 0.5 ml/100g intravenously for four days, the 2,3-DPG level in hemoglobin was $28.59\pm0.38$, while it was $23.20\pm0.33$ ($\mu M/ml$) in the normal saline control group. An increase in the 2,3-DPG level of hemoglobin will promote the release of oxygen from hemoglobin to tissues, benefiting the ischemic heart.

(4) Effects of SMS on thrombus formation and blood coagulation were studied in rabbits in vivo. Doctors gave SMS intravenously at a dose of 2 ml/kg and used normal saline solution as the control.

Within the SMS group, thrombus formation time, prothrombin time and prothrombin comsumption time were all prolonged, and the plasma fibrinogen level decreased, but there was no obvious change in ADP-induced platelet aggregation and thrombin and euglobulinolysis times. These results suggest that SMS inhibits blood coagulation to some extent.

### 3. Codonopsis Pilosula-Astragalus Injection

Liao Jiazhen and Dai Ruihong, et al., observed the effects of Codonopsis Pilosula-Astragalus Injection (CP-A)·on heart failure. It contains 0.5 g each of crude *Radix Codonopsis Pilosulae* and *Radix Astragali* for each ml.

They treated 39 patients with chronic congestive heart failure caused by various heart diseases with CP-A. Eight of these patients underwent cardiac hemodynamic monitoring for 72 hours using Swan-Ganz's catheter to measure the cardiac hemodynamic changes following treatment with CP-A and other control agents.

The results indicated that *Radix Codonopsis Pilosulae* and *Radix Astragali* had a positive inotropic effect on the heart, obviously improving cardiac performance. However, *Radix Salviae Miltirrhizae* did not show such an effect, though it did improve blood viscosity and platelet aggregation more than CP-A.

Doctors also gave 15 patients with angina pectoris (CHD) and 14 with acute myocardial infarction (AMI) CP-A intravenously at a dose of 20 ml. One hour before and one hour after administering medication, they measured systolic time intervals (STI). Meanwhile, they gave Cedilanid-D (0.6 mg i.v.) and 10 percent dextrose (20 ml) as the control groups.

After treatment with CP-A, PEP/LVET levels were reduced from $0.44\pm0.03$ to $0.40\pm0.07$ in patients with CHD and from $0.53\pm0.04$ to $0.49\pm0.03$ in patients with AMI. In patients treated with Cedilanid-D, PEP/LVET levels were reduced from $0.48\pm0.03$ to $0.43\pm0.02$, while the patients who received dextrose experienced no change in their PEP/LVET levels.

Pharmacological studies on the mechanisms of CP-A yielded the following findings:

1) CP-A had no influence on ($Na^+ - K^+$) ATPase activity in rat's myocardial cell membranes in vitro. This suggest that the positive inotropic action of CP-A may not be mediated through inhibition of the sodium pump, as is the case with digitalis glycosides.

2) The activity of cAMP-PDE was inhibited by CP-A, showing a dose-dependant pattern. The cAMP level in myocardiac cells was also enhanced by CP-A from $0.28 \pm 0.24$ pmole/mg wet-cardiac muscle to $1.63 \pm 0.29$ pmole/mg wet-cardiac muscle. It appears that the positive inotropic response to CP-A is associated with significant inhibition of cAMP-PDE activity, leading to an increase of the cAMP level in cardiac cells. Thus, CP-A is a type of nondigitalis cardiotonic.

3) *Radix Codonopsis Pilosulae* and *Radix Astragali* at the concentrations of 0.1-0.8 ml/10ml infusion solution caused dose-dependant increases in papillary muscle-developed tension.

4) CPA caused significant increase in the volume of nutritious blood flow (20.4-37.8 percent in the CP-A group, compared to 49.36 percent in the Isoprenalin group and a decrease of 23.18 percent in the Pituitrium-treated mice) as compared with that of the Tween-80 control.

5) ADP induced platelet aggregation was inhibited by CP-A at a rate of $55.1 \pm 9.6$ percent.

6) The cAMP and cGMP levels of platelets were increased by CP-A, whereas no significant change was observed in the dextrose control group. The results of experiments in vitro also revealed a significant increase in the cAMP and cGMP levels in platelet in response to CP-A. According to the current hypothesis, an increase in platelet aggregation in correlated to a decrease in cAMP level in platelet. The results of the present study suggest that inhibition of platelet aggregation by CP-A may be mediated by increasing the cAMP level in platelet.

7) The platelet PDE activity was reduced by CP-A, which may be partly responsible for the increase in cyclic nucleotide levels.

8) The activity of CaM (calmodulin) was inhibited by CP-A, suggesting that the decreased activity of PDE caused by CP-A in platelet is partly due to CPA inhibiting CaM, an effect similar to milrinone, a non-digitalis glycoside.

# CHAPTER XXVI   SHOCK

Shock is a complex clinical state in which cardiac output is insufficient for tissue and cell requirements, resulting in reduced tissue perfusion and therefore tissue hypoxia and accumulation of metabolites.

Patients in shock are usually hypotensive with a systolic arterial pressure of 90 mmHg or less. They have cold, clammy, cyanotic skin, thready rapid pulse and dulled sensorium, or they are confused and oliguric. These symptoms occur in addition to those of the underlying, precipitating disease.

The major causes of shock are reduced venous return, as in hemorrhage, dehydration and endotoxin shock, and reduced cardiac output, as the cardiogenic shock in myocardial infarction and myocarditis.

In traditional Chinese medicine, shock falls under the category of either "*Jue* syndrome" (syndrome of temporary loss of consciousness) or "*Tuo* syndrome" (collapse syndrome).

## ETIOLOGY AND PATHOGENESIS

### 1. Invasion of pathogenic heat
Pathogenic heat damages primary *qi* and consumes body fluids, leading to exhaustion of *qi* and *yin*. Furthermore, overabundant pathogenic heat may penetrate the pericardium and disturb the mind, followed by impairment of consciousness. Endotoxic shock can be included in this category.

### 2. Exhaustion of *yang-qi*
Shock may occur in severe or protracted illnesses which exhaust the primary *qi*, or because of an overabundance of *yin*-cold in the interior, which consumes *yang-qi*.

### 3. Exhaustion of *yin*-essence
Severe bleeding, diarrhea, vomiting and sweating may result in cases where *yin*-essence is exhausted. Exhausted *yin*-essence will cause *yin* and *yang* to separate.

## DIFFERENTIAL DIAGNOSIS OF SYNDROMES

Primary manifestations: Deadly cold limbs, excessive cold sweating, pale complexion, shortness of breath, listlessness or loss of consciousness, cyanosis, pale and purplish tongue and deep, feeble, hardly perceptible pulse.

*Jue* syndrome and *tuo* syndrome share these symptoms. In addition, these syndromes can be further categorized as follows:

1. Heat-*jue* occurs in an infectious disease, accompanied by fever, thirst, irritability, yellowish urine, constipation, reddened tongue with yellow coating and rapid pulse.

2. Cold-*jue* is characterized by a sudden onset and is not preceded by fever but with

the symptoms of the underlying disease.

The distinguishing feature of *jue* syndrome is a pronounced coldness of the extremities associated with the clinical manifestations of the underlying disease. In general, *jue* syndrome is considered early shock, *tuo* syndrome advanced shock.

3. *Yang-tuo* is similar to cold-*jue* in clinical manifestations, but they are more severe.

4. *Yin-tuo* is caused by severe exhaustion of *yin* essence, so it usually occurs after serious hemorrhage, diarrhea and/or vomiting and excessive profuse sweating.

*Tuo*-syndrome corresponds to severe shock. Septic shock may be included under heat-*jue* and other types of shock under cold-*jue*. Hemorrhagic or hypovolumic shock and shock in burns belong to the *yin-tuo* syndrome; other types of shock, such as cardiogenic shock and anaphylaxis shocks, are considered *yang-tuo* syndromes. Finally, it should be pointed out that the classification of shock in traditional Chinese medicine is not without controversy.

## TREATMENT

### 1. Heat-*jue*

Principle of treatment: Invigorate primary *qi* and expel pathogenic factors.

Formula of choice: Huanglian Jiedu Tang (Antidotal Decoction of Coptis) and Shengmai San (Pulse-activating Powder).

### 2. Cold-*jue* or *yang-tuo*

Principle of treatment: Recuperate depleted *yang* and rescue the patient from collapse.

Formula of choice: Shen Fu Tang (Decoction of Ginseng and Aconite), Prepared Aconite Decoction and Qi Fu Tang (Decoction of Astragalus and Prepared Aconite); in these recipes, Ginseng and Astragalus replenish primary *qi*; Prepared Aconite recuperates depleted *yang*.

### 3. *Yin-tuo*

Principle of treatment: Replenish *qi*, recuperate depleted *yang* and nourish *yin*.

Formula of choice: Shengmai San (Pulse-activating Powder) and Prepared Aconite.

Acupuncture treatment

Primary acupoints: Shuigou (GV 26), Baihui (GV 20), Neiguan (PC 6), Qihai (CV 6), Zusanli (ST 36), Hegu (LI 4) and Taichong (LR 3).

Shuigou, Baihui and Neiguan are points for resuscitation; Qihai and Zusanli replenish *qi* and recuperate *yang*; Hegu and Taichong regulate the circulation of *qi* and blood. Practitioners should use these points with the reinforcing method and may combine them with moxibustion to warm *yang*.

## MODERN RESEARCH

Sheng Mai San (Pulse-activating Powder) is a famous prescription for treating both *qi* and *yin* deficiency. Nowadays it is prepared as an injection (Sheng Mai Injection, or SMI) for intravenous administration. Ten ml of SMI contains *Radix Ginseng* (1 g), *Radix Ophiopogonis* (3.21 g) and *Fructus Schizandrae* (1.56 g).

Doctors at Tianjin Nan Kai Hospital first used this prescription in 1972 to treat patients with cardiogenic shock caused by acute myocardial infarction. The positive results obtained there have prompted doctors throughout China to use SMI in treating various types of shock.

The usual intravenous dose is 10-20 ml SMI mixed with 20 ml of 10 percent to 25 percent dextrose given slowly, to be repeated as needed to maintain blood pressure. SMI is safe for clinical use without obvious side effects. However, large doses or high concentrations and rapid intravenous injection should be avoided because they may cause a fall in blood pressure and depression of the heart function.

Extensive clinical experiences attest to the efficacy of SMI. For example, a report on 103 cases of acute myocardial infarction complicated with cardiogenic shock showed that the mortality rate from shock in the group treated with Western medicine alone was 52 percent, whereas in the group treated by SMI and Western medicine the rate was 25 percent. Fuwai Hospital reported that among 87 patients with acute myocardial infarction complicated with cardiogenic shock, the mortality rate was 40 percent in the 48 cases treated only with Western medicine, whereas in the 34 cases treated with SMI and Western medicine the mortality rate was 18.6 percent. Sichuan Medical College studied 114 cases of various types of shock treated with SMI and found that it elevated blood pressure within five minutes to one hour and steadily sustained it for an average of 17.3 hours.

After the injection, doctors noted a mild increase in blood pressure, though the extreme coldness of the limbs and cyanosis were alleviated in about an hour, indicating improvement in peripheral microcirculation. In some shock patients whose blood pressure could not be stably sustained by either Western or Chinese drugs alone, the combination of a vasopressor agent and SMI proved efficacious.

SMI used with such Western medicines as dopamine and aramine can exhibit the following coordinated actions: strengthening the vasopressor's effect of raising blood pressure and reducing the dosage of the vasopressor and decreasing its side effects so that the prognosis of shock improves.

In pharmacological studies, Sheng Mai San has been found to strengthen the heart function, lower the oxygen consumption of the myocardium, increase the blood flow of the coronary artery, improve myocardial metabolism and correct various forms of experimental shock.

Doctors at Tianjin Nankai Hospital studied the effects of Sheng Mai San on hemorrhagic shock induced in dogs by bleeding them until their systolic pressure reached 20 mmHg. The animals then received an injection of Sheng Mai San (SMI). Their blood pressure rose to $59.0\pm13.5$ mmHg. Dogs injected with normal saline solution showed no effects, their systolic pressure being $9.0\pm14.0$ mmHg. Similar results were obtained in rabbits after they had been bled to a level of 30 mmHg arterial pressure. Their blood pressure rose to 82 mmHg after SMI, and the effect persisted for about one hour.

Researchers at Beijing Medical University observed the effects of Sheng Mai San on the mesenteric microcirculation of shock induced by ligating the mesenteric artery in rabbits. Mesenteric vascular constriction occurred in only two of 10 rabbits in the Sheng Mai Injection group. Disturbance of microcirculation diminished and the mortality rate decreased markedly in the treated group compared with the control group.

Doctors also studied the effects of Sheng Mai Injection on shock induced by the endotoxin of *B. dysenteriae* in mice. The results showed that the mortality in the SMI group was half that of the control group. Further experiments revealed that SMI could reduce capillary permeability and antagonize the inhibitory effect of the endotoxin on the phagocytosis of the reticuloendothelial system.

Physicians at the Fourth Military Medical University researched the effect of Sheng Mai Injection on the prevention and treatment of experimental burn shock in dogs. Dogs with burns over 25 percent of their body surface were randomly divided into three groups: one group received 10 percent glucose solution, another group solution No. 62 (consisting of NaCl [8 g], KCl [0.075 g], $CaCl_2$ [0.1 g], Dolantin [0.05 g] and Procain [0.5 g] in 1000 ml) and the third group SMI. Physicians defined shock as a fall of systolic arterial pressure to a level below 80 mmHg. In the SMI group, the period between burn and the onset of shock was $16.83\pm3.65$ hours, much longer than the $6.47\pm2.23$ hours in the glucose group and the $12.81\pm3.61$ hours in the solution No. 62 group.

Doctors also found that the volume of urine increased significantly in the SMI group compared with the other groups. The hematocrit in the control group increased significantly eight hours after the burns, whereas it returned to normal over this period of time in the SMI group.

## 2. Restoring Depleted *Yang* and Rescuing the Patient from Collapse

Researchers have also studied the pharmacological actions of Shen Fu Tang in animal experiments on cardiovascular activities under normal and shock conditions. They used refined preparation of the product composed of *Radix Aconiti Praeparata* (0.5 g/ml) and Ginsenosides (2.4 mg/ml). Its $LD_{50}$ was 11.2 ml/kg i.v.

Shen Fu Tang increased the blood flow of the coronary artery in an isolated rabbit heart by $54.5\pm7.9$ percent at 0.03 ml/kg; it also strengthened heart contractions, but there was no change in the heart rate.

Shen Fu Qing Injection (SFQI) has proven another effective treatment for shock. This recipe is composed of *Radix Ginseng, Radix Aconiti Praeparata* and *Pericarpium Citri Reticulatae Viride*. Of the 30 cases of septic shock doctors treated with Shen Fu Qing Injection, 15 recovered from shock in an average of 26.5 hours, eight showed improvement and seven did not respond. Improvement in hypotension began in three minutes to three hours, with an average of 86 minutes. The systolic blood pressure increased by an average of 41.6 mmHg and the diastolic pressure by an average of 27.1 mmHg.

Pharmacological experiments using SFQI on endotoxin shock in Wistar rats showed that immediately after an intravenous injection of endotoxin (lipopolysaccharide Oss Br of B. Coli) 4 mg/kg, the group of rats receiving SFQI retained their blood pressure at $104.8\pm16.3$ mmHg, compared with $72.3\pm16.6$ mmHg in the control group.

Ninety minutes after injection of the endotoxin, it was found that the mesenteric arteriole lumen was $15.27\pm2.65$ μM in the SFQI group, compared with $12.08\pm2.57$ μM in the control group. These findings indicate that SFQI inhibits the constriction of the mesenteric arteriole caused by endotoxin.

It also appears that the action of *Pericarpium Citri Reticulatae Viride* (green orange peel) is quite similar to that of α-receptor agonists, since its actions are antagonized by regitine, an α-receptor inhibitor. The action of aconitine (the pure alkaloid of aconiti) is similar to that of ß-receptor agonists, as it is antagonized by practolol, a ß-receptor inhibitor.

Pharmacologists also observed the protective effects of Si Ni Tang on endotoxin shock. An intravenous dose of 8-10 mg/kg of *B. Coli* 055 B5 endotoxin in rabbits caused the carotid arterial pressure to fall to a level of 50-70 mmHg. Forty minutes after injection of Si Ni Tang, the carotid arterial pressure increased; meanwhile, the bulbar conjunctive microcirculation improved and the time required for red blood cell electrophoresis shortened. The contraction of the heart was strengthened and the coronary artery blood flow of the isolated heart also increased. All these parameters when compared with those of the control group were statistically significant.

Researchers also treated experimental hemorrhagic shock with Si Ni Tang. Eight rabbits with hemorrhagic shock received the recipe administered via the duodenal fistula through a fixed tube at a dose of 40 ml. All eight rabbits survived, as compared with four deaths among the eight rabbits in the saline control group.

Si Ni Tang also lessened the shock induced by superior mesenteric arterial occlusion. Doctors divided 40 experimental animals randomly into four groups: Group A received only one dose of Si Ni Tang; Group B received the same recipe regularly for two weeks; groups C and D served as controls and received normal saline in the same dosage patterns as groups A and B. The death rates in Groups A and B were 30 percent and 20 percent, respectively, and 70 percent in the control groups. Autopsies of the experimental animals showed that in the treated group the colour of the mucous membrane of the small intestine was red with few bleeding spots and no large areas of necrosis, whereas in the control group the colour of the mucous membrane of the small intestine was darkened with disseminated bleeding, multiple ulcers and necrosis.

### 3. The Principle of Replenishing *Qi* and Promoting Blood Circulation

It is well known that disseminated intravascular coagulation (DIC) is a serious complication of shock with a very high mortality rate. However, doctors successfully treated 22 cases of shock complicated with DIC with Chinese drugs for replenishing *qi* and promoting blood flow, with a survival rate of 72.7 percent. They found that drugs for promoting blood circulation given in the early stage of shock could prevent or diminish DIC, leading to a lower mortality rate from shock.

There are numerous herbal drugs for replenishing *qi* and blood circulation. Researchers used Decoction for Replenishing *Qi* and Promoting Blood Flow (consisting of *Radix Astragali, Radix Salviae Miltiorrhizae, Radix Angelicae Sinensis, Rhizoma Ligustici* and *Herba Leonuri*) in an experimental study of endotoxin shock in rabbits.

The mortality rate in the treated group was 32.3 percent and 67.7 percent in the control group. Compared with the control group, the plasma level of fibrinogen and the Euglobuline solution time in the treated group were reduced significantly, at 15 and 60 minutes, respectively, after injection of the herbal drugs. The thrombin and recalcification times were prolonged, and the hypotension caused by endotoxin was also diminished.

## 4. Purgating Heat and Detoxification

Septic shock is caused by systemic infection and bacterial endotoxin, which corresponds to the traditional Chinese medicine concept that epidemic toxic heat causes the collapse syndrome (*jue-tuo* syndrome). Obviously, antibiotics have no effect on the toxin, although they do possess antibacterial action. Experimental studies on animals have shown that certain Chinese medicinal herbs can clear away fever and toxins. Among these are *Radix Isatidis*, *Herba Taraxaci*, *Herba Andrographitis* and *Radix Scrophulariae*. They stimulate the nonspecific immune functions of the body, reduce the visceral damages induced by endotoxin and antagonize the endotoxin to some extent.

Doctors at Tongji Medical University reported on the effect of "Injection to Eliminate Heat Toxin" (Re Du Qing Injection, or RDQ, composed of *Flos Lonicerae*, *Herba Taraxaci*, *Folium Isatidis* and *Herba Houttuyniae* on DIC. The DIC model was produced by injecting the endotoxin of *Escherichia Coli* into rabbits. The results showed that the hematological changes of DIC in the dexamethasone and RDQ groups were markedly diminished compared with those of the saline control group.

Morphological observation by means of electron microscope also demonstrated the anti-DIC action of these herbs. The incidence of DIC was 25 percent in the RDQ group compared with 83.3 percent in the saline control group. The formation of fibrin microthrombus in glomerulus was also significantly reduced in the RDQ group. Observation of the ultrastructure of the glomerular endothelial cells and hepatic cells under an electron microscope showed that damage in the RDQ group was milder than that noted in the saline control group.

Pharmacological studies of the effects of rhubarb on an experimental infection in rabbits revealed that it could increase the level of prostaglandin E (PGE) in the cerebrospinal fluid drained from the third ventricle. There was also a positive correlation between PGE and anal temperature, suggesting that the action of rhubarb might be mediated by PGE. The phagocytic function and the level of total serum complement were also increased following administration of the purgative mixture. This suggests that purgation can improve the resistance of the host.

## 5. The effect of *Fructus Aurantii Immaturus*

In 1973, doctors found that the extract of *Fructus Aurantii Immaturus* (FAI) increased blood pressure in anesthetized animals as effectively as neosynephrine and surpassed neosynephrine in terms of producing a more prolonged rise in blood pressure. FAI also caused an increase in the pulse, a decrease in the arrhythmias or reflex bradycardia and an increase in the blood perfusion in the heart, brain and kidneys. In a clinical study of 94 cases of various types of shock (including 49 cases of septic shock and 14 cases of cardiogenic shock) treated with FAI and no other vasoactive agents, 70 cases responded favourably to FAI, with a rise in blood pressure within 30 minutes to a level of 90 mmHg or more. At same time, the heart sounds become louder, the pulse stronger, the limbs warmer and the volume of urine greater in these patients. Pharmacologists discovered that FAI contained neosynephrine as one of its constituents.

# APPENDIX

# SELECTED FORMULAE AND PATENT (READY-TO-USE) MEDICINES

Baihe Gujin Tang ( 百合固金汤 ) Lily Decoction for Strengthening the Lungs
*Radix Rehmanniae* (dried rehmannia root 生地黄 *Shengdihuang*) 6g
*Radix Rehmanniae Praeparata* (prepared rehmannia root 熟地黄 *shudihuang*) 9g
*Radix Ophiopogonis* (ophiopogon root 麦冬 *maidong*) 5g
*Bulbus Lilli* (lily bulb 百合 *baihe*) 3g
*Radix Paeoniae Alba* (white peony root 白芍 *baishao*) 3g
*Radix Angelicae Sinensis* (Chinese angelica root 当归 *danggui*) 3g
*Bulbus Fritillariae* (fritillary bulb 贝母 *beimu*) 3g
*Radix Glycyrrhizae* (liquorice 甘草 *gancao*) 3g
*Radix Scrophulariae* (scrophularia root 玄参 *xuanshen*) 2g
*Radix Platycodi* (platycodon root 桔梗 *jiegeng*) 2g
Actions: Nourish *yin*, remove heat, moisten the lungs and resolve phlegm.
Indications: Deficiency of *yin* of the lungs and kidneys with exuberant fire manifested as sore throat, cough and shortness of breath, blood-stained sputum, heat sensation in the palms and soles, reddened tongue with little coating and thready, rapid pulse.

Baihu Tang ( 白虎汤 ) White Tiger Decoction
*Rhizoma Anemarrhenae* (anemarrhena rhizome 知母 *zhimu*) 9g
*Gypsum Fibrosum* (gypsum 石膏 *shigao*) 30g
*Radix Glycyrrhizae* (liquorice 甘草 *gancao*) 3g
*Semen Oryzae Nonglutinosae* (nonglutinous rice 粳米 *jingmi*) 9g
Actions: Clear heat and promote production of body fluids.
Indications: High fever with flushed face, thirst, sweating, dry, yellow tongue coating, and gigantic pulse; also for diabetes involving the middle-*jiao*.

Banxia Baizhu Tianma Tang ( 半夏白术天麻汤 ) Decoction of Pinellia, White Atractylodes and Gastrodia
*Rhizoma Pinelliae* (pinellia tuber 半夏 *banxia*) 9g
*Rhizoma Gastrodiae* (gastrodia tuber 天麻 *tianma*) 6g
Poria (poria 茯苓 *fuling*) 6g
*Exocarpium Citri Reticulatae* (red tangerine peel 橘红 *juhong*) 6g
*Rhizoma Atractylodis Macrocephalae* (white atractylodes rhizome 白术 *baizhu*) 9g
*Radix Glycyrrhizae* (liquorice 甘草 *gancao*) 2g
Actions: Resolve wind-phlegm and reinforce the spleen.
Indications: Upward invasion of wind-phlegm manifested by dizziness and headache associated with stuffiness in the chest, white greasy tongue coating and taut, slippery pulse.

Banxia Xiexin Tang ( 半夏泻心汤 ) Pinellia Decoction for Purging Stomach Fire
*Rhizoma Pinelliae* (pinellia tuber 半夏 *banxia*) 12g
*Radix Scutellariae* (scutellaria root 黄芩 *huangqin*) 9g

*Rhizoma Zingiberis* (dried ginger  干姜  *ganjiang*) 9g
*Radix Ginseng* (ginseng  人参  *renshen*) 9g
*Radix Glycyrrhizae Praeparata* (prepared liquorice 炙甘草 *zhigancao*) 6g
*Rhizoma Coptidis* (coptis root  黄连  *huanglian*) 3g
*Fructus Ziziphi Jujubae* (Chinese date  大枣  *dazao*) 4pcs
Actions: Regulate the stomach function.
Indications: Painless stuffiness, retching or vomiting due to dysfunction of the stomach.

Baohe Wan (  保和丸  ) Lenitive Pill
*Fructus Crataegi* (charred hawthorn fruit  焦山楂  *jiaoshanzha*) 300g
*Massa Fermentata Medicinalis* (medicated leaven  神曲  *shenqu*) 100g
*Rhizoma Pinelliae* (prepared pinellia tuber  制半夏  *zhibanxia*) 100g
Poria (poria  茯苓  *fuling*) 100g
*Pericarpium Citri Reticulatae* (tangerine peel  陈皮  *chenpi*) 50g
*Fructus Forsythiae* (forsythia fruit  连翘  *lianqiao*) 50g
*Semen Raphani* (radish seed  莱菔子  *laifuzi*) 50g
*Fructus Hordei Germinatus* (germinated barley  麦芽  *maiya*) 50g
Mixed, pulverized and made into pills, 6-9g for each dose.
Actions: Promotes digestion.
Indications: Indigestion.

Bazheng San (  八正散  ) All-orientation Health-restoring Powder
*Caulis Clematidis Armandii* (Sichuan clematis stem  木通  *mutong*)
*Herba Dianthi* (Chinese pink herb  瞿麦  *qumai*)
*Semen Plantaginis* (plantain seed  车前子  *cheqianzi*)
*Herba Polygoni Avicularis* (common knotgrass  萹蓄  *bianxu*)
*Talcum* (talc  滑石  *huashi*)
*Radix Glycyrrhizae* (liquorice  甘草  *gancao*)
*Radix et Rhizoma Rhei* (rhubarb  大黄  *dahuang*)
*Fructus Gardeniae* (capejasmine fruit  栀子  *zhizi*)
Mix equal quantities and make into powder, 6g for each dose.
Actions: Remove heat, induce diuresis and relieve stranguria.
Indications: Damp-heat in the urinary bladder.

Bazhen Tang (  八珍汤  ) Decoction of Eight Precious Ingredients
*Radix Angelicae Sinensis* (Chinese angelica root  当归  *danggui*) 9g
*Radix Ginseng* (ginseng  人参  *renshen*) 9g
*Radix Paeoniae Alba* (white peony root  白芍  *baishao*) 9g
*Rhizoma Atractylodis Macrocephalae* (white atractylodes rhizome  白术  *baizhu*) 9g
Poria (poria  茯苓  *fuling*) 9g
*Radix Rehmanniae Praeparata* (prepared rehmannia root  熟地黄  *shudihuang*) 12g
*Rhizoma Ligustici Chuanxiong* (chuanxiong rhizome  川芎  *chuanxiong*) 6g
*Radix Glycyrrhizae Praeparata* (prepared liquorice  炙甘草  *zhigancao*) 3g
Actions: Replenish *qi* and blood.
Indications: Deficiency of both *qi* and blood.

**Bufei Tang** ( 补肺汤 ) Lung-tonifying Decoction

*Radix Ginseng* (ginseng 人参 *renshen*) 9g

*Radix Astragali* (astragalus root 黄芪 *huangqi*) 24g

*Radix Rehmanniae Praeparata* (prepared rehmannia root 熟地黄 *shudihuang*) 24g

*Fructus Schisandrae* (schisandra fruit 五味子 *wuweizi*) 6g

*Radix Asteris* (aster root 紫菀 *ziyuan*) 9g

*Cortex Mori Radicis* (mulberry bark 桑白皮 *sangbaipi*) 12g

Actions: Replenish the lung-*qi* and relieve cough.

Indications: Cough, shortness of breath and spontaneous sweating due to deficiency of lung *qi*.

**Bugan Tang** ( 补肝汤 ) Decoction for Replenishing the Liver

*Radix Angelicae Sinensis* (Chinese angelica root 当归 *danggui*) 9g

*Rhizoma Ligustici Chuanxiong* (chuanxiong rhizome 川芎 *chuanxiong*) 6g

*Radix Paeoniae* (peony root 芍药 *shaoyao*) 9g

*Radix Rehmanniae Praeparata* (prepared rehmannia root 熟地黄 *shudihuang*) 15g

*Semen Ziziphae Spinosae* (wild jujuba seed 酸枣仁 *suanzaoren*) 9g

*Radix Glycyrrhizae Praeparata* (prepared liquorice 炙甘草 *zhigancao*) 3g

*Fructus Chaenomelis* (chaenomeles fruit 木瓜 *mugua*) 9g

Actions: Nourish *yin*-blood of the liver.

Indications: Headache, veritgo, tinnitus and tremor or numbness of limbs due to deficiency of *yin*-blood of the liver.

**Buyang Huanwu Tang** ( 补阳还五汤 ) Decoction for Invigorating *Yang* and Recuperation

*Radix Astragali* (astragalus root 黄芪 *huangqi*) 30g

*Radix Angelicae Sinensis* (Chinese angelica root 当归 *danggui*) 9g

*Radix Paeoniae Rubra* (red peony root 赤芍 *chishao*) 9g

*Lumbricus* (earthworm 地龙 *dilong*) 9g

*Rhizoma Ligustici Chuanxiong* (chuanxiong rhizome 川芎 *chuanxiong*) 6g

*Semen Persicae* (peach kernal 桃仁 *taoren*) 9g

*Flos Carthami* (safflower 红花 *honghua*) 9g

Actions: Replenish *qi* and activate blood circulation in collaterals.

Indications: Sequelae of apoplexy.

**Buzhong Yiqi Tang** ( 补中益气汤 ) Decoction for Reinforcing Middle-*jiao* and Replenishing *Qi*

*Radix Astragali* (astragalus root 黄芪 *huangqi*) 15g

*Radix Glycyrrhizae Praeparata* (prepared liquorice 炙甘草 *zhigancao*) 5g

*Radix Ginseng* (ginseng 人参 *renshen*) 9g

*Radix Angelicae Sinensis* (Chinese angelica root 当归 *danggui*) 9g

*Pericarpium Citri Reticulatae* (tangerine peel 陈皮 *chenpi*) 6g

*Rhizoma Cimicifugae* (cimicifuga rhizome 升麻 *shengma*) 3g

*Radix Bupleuri* (bupleurum root 柴胡 *chaihu*) 3g

*Rhizoma Atractylodis Macrocephalae* (white atractylodes rhizome 白术 *baizhu*) 9g

Actions: Replenish *qi* of the spleen and stomach and elevate *qi* of the middle-*jiao*.

Indications: Syndromes due to deficiency of *qi* of the spleen and stomach and hysteroptosis or gastroptosis due to deficiency of *qi* of the middle-*jiao*.

**Chaihu Shugan San** ( 柴胡疏肝散 ) Bupleurum Powder for Soothing the Liver
  *Radix Bupleuri* (bupleurum root 柴胡 *chaihu*) 6g
  *Pericarpium Citri Reticulatae* (tangerine peel 陈皮 *chenpi*) 6g
  *Fructus Aurantii* (bitter orange 枳壳 *zhiqiao*) 6g
  *Radix Paeoniae Alba* (white peony root 白芍 *baishao*) 9g
  *Radix Glycyrrhizae Praeparata* (prepared liquorice 炙甘草 *zhigancao*) 3g
  *Rhizoma Cyperi* (cyperus tuber 香附 *xiangfu*) 6g
  *Rhizoma Ligustici Chuanxiong* (chuanxiong rhizome 川芎 *chuanxiong*) 6g
  Actions: Promote the flow of liver *qi* and blood and relieve pain.
  Indications: Pain in the hypochondriac region with alternate spells of fever and chills
  due to stagnancy of liver *qi*.

**Chixiaodou Danggui San** ( 赤小豆当归散 )    Powder of Phaseolus Seeds and Chinese
Angelica  Root
  *Semen Phaseoli* (red phaseolus bean 赤小豆 *chixiaodou*) 30g
  *Radix Angelicae Sinensis* (Chinese angelica root 当归 *danggui*) 15g
  Mixed and pulverized, 9g for each dose.
  Actions: Reduce heat and regulate blood flow.
  Indications: Bloody stool due to heat in the large intestine.

**Da Buyin Wan** ( 大补阴丸 ) Bolus for Replenshing *Yin*
  *Cortex Phellodendri* (phellodendron bark 黄柏 *huangbai*) 80g
  *Rhizoma Anemarrhenae* (anemarrhena rhizome 知母 *zhimu*) 80g
  *Radix Rehmanniae Praeparata* (prepared rehmannia root 熟地黄 *shudihuang*) 120g
  *Plastrum Testudinis* (tortoise plastron 龟板 *guiban*) 120g
  *Medulla Spinalis Suis* (spinal cord of swine 猪脊髓 *zhujisui*) 160g
  Mixed equal quantities of each pulverized and make into pills, 6g 2-3 times daily.
  Actions: Replenish *yin* of the liver and kidneys.
  Indications: Hectic fever and night sweating due to flaring up of fire caused by
  deficiency of *yin* of the liver and kidneys.

**Da Bu Yuan Jian** ( 大补元煎 ) Potent Decoction for Replenishing Original Essence
  *Radix Ginseng* (ginseng 人参 *renshen*) 3-9g
  *Rhizoma Dioscoreae* (Chinese yam 山药 *shanyao*) 6g
  *Radix Rehmanniae Praeparata* (prepared rehmannia root 熟地黄 *shudihuang*) 9-30g
  *Cortex Eucommiae* (eucommia bark 杜仲 *duzhong*) 6g
  *Radix Angelicae Sinensis* (Chinese angelica root 当归 *danggui*) 6g
  *Fructus Corni* (dogwood fruit 山茱萸 *shanzhuyu*) 3g
  *Fructus Lycii* (wolfberry fruit 枸杞子 *gouqizi*) 6g
  *Radix Glycyrrhizae Praeparata* (prepared liquorice 炙甘草 *zhigancao*) 3g
  Actions: Replenish *yin*, blood and *qi*.
  Indications: Serious deficiency of kidney essence, *qi* and blood.

**Da Chaihu Tang** ( 大柴胡汤 ) Major Bupleurum Decoction
  *Radix Bupleuri* (bupleurum root 柴胡 *chaihu*) 9g
  *Radix Scutellariae* (scutellaria root 黄芩 *huangqin*) 9g

*Radix Paeoniae Alba* (white peony root  白芍  *baishao*) 9g

*Rhizoma Pinelliae* (pinellia tuber  半夏  *banxia*) 9g

*Fructus Aurantii Immaturus* (immature bitter orange  枳实  *zhishi*) 9g

*Radix et Rhizoma Rhei* (rhubarb  大黄  *dahuang*) 6g

*Fructus Ziziphi Jujubae* (Chinese date  大枣  *dazao*) 4pcs

*Rhizoma Zingiberis Recens* (fresh ginger  生姜  *shengjiang*) 12g

Actions: Treat *shaoyang* disease and purge away accumulated heat.

Indications: Acute cholecystitis, cholelithiasis and acute pancreatitis.

**Danggui Buxue Tang** (  当归补血汤  ) Chinese Angelica Decoction for Replenishing Blood

*Radix Astragali* (astragalus root  黄芪  *huangqi*) 30g

*Radix Angelicae Sinensis* (Chinese angelica root  当归  *danggui*) 6g

Actions: Replenish *qi* and promote production of blood.

Indications: Deficiency of blood and fever due to deficiency of blood.

**Daochi San** (  导赤散  ) Powder for Treating Dark Urine

*Radix Rehmanniae* (dried rehmannia root  生地黄  *shengdihuang*)

*Radix Glycyrrhizae* (liquorice  甘草  *gancao*)

*Caulis Clematidis Armandii* (Sichuan clematis stem  木通  *mutong*)

*Herba Lophatheri* (lophatherum  竹叶  *zhuye*)

Actions: Clear the heart of excess fire and induce diuresis.

Indications: Hyperactivity of heart fire manifested as thirst, fidgetiness, ulcer of the tongue, burning pain in the urethra during micturition and passage of dark urine.

**Dingchuan Tang** (  定喘汤  ) Antiasthmatic Decoction

*Semen Ginkgo* (ginkgo seed  白果  *baiguo*) 9g

*Herba Ephedrae* (ephedra  麻黄  *mahuang*) 9g

*Fructus Perillae* (perilla seed  紫苏子  *zisuzi*) 6g

*Radix Glycyrrhizae* (liquorice  甘草  *gancao*) 3g

*Flos Farfarae* (coltsfoot flower  款冬花  *kuandonghua*) 9g

*Semen Armeniacae Amarum* (bitter apricot kernal  苦杏仁  *kuxingren*) 5g

*Cortex Mori Radicis* (mulberry bark  桑白皮  *sangbaipi*) 9g

*Radix Scutellariae* (scutellaria root  黄芩  *huangqin*) 5g

*Rhizoma Pinelliae* (pinelliae tuber  半夏  *banxia*) 9g

Actions: Relieve asthma and resolve phlegm.

*Indications*: Asthma with accumulaton of heat and phlegm after exposure to wind and cold.

**Diyu San** (  地榆散  ) Sanguisorba Powder

*Radix Sanguisorbae* (sanguisorba root  地榆  *diyu*) 15g

*Radix Rubiae* (rubia root  茜草  *qiancao*) 15g

*Radix Scutellariae* (scutellaria root  黄芩  *huangqin*) 15g

*Rhizoma Coptidis* (coptis root  黄连  *huanglian*) 15g

*Fructus Gardeniae* (capejasmine fruit  栀子  *zhizi*) 10g

Poria (poria  茯苓  *fuling*) 15g

Mixed and pulverized, 9g for each dose.

Actions: Arrest bleeding by cooling blood.

Indications: Hematochezia caused by damp-heat.

**Duqi Wan** ( 都气丸 ) Dyspnea-relieving Pill

*Radix Rehmanniae Praeparata* (prepared rehmannia root  熟地黄  *shudihuang*) 240g

*Fructus Corni* (dogwood fruit 山茱萸  *shanzhuyu*) 120g

*Rhizoma Dioscoreae* (Chinese yam  山药  *shanyao*) 120g

*Rhizoma Alismatis* (alismatis rhizome  泽泻 *zexie*) 90g

*Cortex Moutan Radicis* (moutan bark  牡丹皮  *mudanpi*) 90g

Poria (poria 茯苓 *fuling*) 90g

*Fructus Schisandrae* (schisandra fruit  五味子  *wuweizi*) 90g

Actions: Tonify the kidneys and restore the kidneys' function in receiving air.

Indications: Dyspnea due to deficiency of kidneys in receiving air.

**Erchen Tang** ( 二陈汤 ) Decoction of Two Old Drugs

*Pericarpium Citri Reticulatae* (tangerine peel  陈皮  *chenpi*) 6g

*Rhizoma Pinelliae* (pinellia tuber 半夏 *banxia*) 6g

Poria (poria 茯苓 *fuling*) 9g

*Radix Glycyrrhizae Praeparata* (prepared liquorice  炙甘草  *zhigancao*) 1.5g

Actions: Remove damp-phlegm and regulate spleen *qi*

Indications: Syndromes of damp-phlegm due to dysfunction of the spleen manifested by cough and expectoration with nausea and stuffy feeling in the chest or by vomiting, dizziness and palpitations.

**Erdong Tang** ( 二冬汤 ) Asparagus and Ophiopogon Decoction

*Radix Asparagi* (asparagus root  天冬  *tiandong*) 8g

*Radix Ophiopogonis* (ophiopogon  麦冬  *maidong*) 9g

*Radix Trichosanthis* (trichosanthes root  天花粉  *tianhuafen*) 3g

*Radix Scutellariae* (scutellaria root  黄芩  *huangqin*) 3g

*Rhizoma Anemarrhenae* (anemarrhena rhizome  知母  *zhimu*) 3g

*Folium Nelumbinis* (lotus leaf  荷叶  *heye*) 3g

*Radix Ginseng* (ginseng  人参  *renshen*) 1.5g

*Radix Glycyrrhizae* (liquorice  甘草  *gancao*) 1.5g

Actions: Relieve dryness-heat of the lungs and stomach.

Indications: Diabetes involving the upper-*jiao*.

**Fugui Lizhong Tang** ( 附桂理中汤 ) Decoction for Regulating Middle-*jiao* with Aconite and Cinnamon

Lizhong Tang (Decoction for Regulating Middle-*jiao*) plus *Radix Aconiti Lateralis Praeparata* (prepared aconite root  附子  *fuzi*) 9g and *Cortex Cinnamomi* (cinnamon bark  肉桂  *rougui*) 6g.

Actions: Warm the spleen and stomach (more potent than Fuzi Lizhong Tang).

Indications: Deficiency-cold syndromes of the spleen and stomach.

**Fuzi Lizhong Tang** ( 附子理中汤 ) Decoction for Regulating Middle-*jiao* with Aconite

Lizhong Tang (Decoction for Regulating Middle-*jiao*) puls *Radix Aconiti Lateralis Praeparata* (prepared aconite root  附子  *fuzi*) 9g

Actions: Warm the spleen and stomach.

Indications: Deficiency-cold syndromes of the spleen and stomach.

Fuzi Tang (　附子汤　) Aconite Decoction
  *Radix Aconiti Lateralis Praeparata* (prepared aconite root　附子　*fuzi*) 12g
  Poria (poria　茯苓　*fuling*) 9g
  *Radix Ginseng* (ginseng　人参　*renshen*) 6g
  *Rhizoma Atractylodis Macrocephalae* (white atractylodes rhizome　白术　*baizhu*) 12g
  *Radix Paeoniae Alba* (white peony root　白芍　*baishao*) 9g
  Actions: Warm the kidneys and remove cold and damp.
  Indications: Syndromes of cold-damp due to deficiency of *yang*, particularly mani-
  fested as general aching and arthralgia.

Ganmao Tuire Chongji (　感冒退热冲剂　) Antipyretic Granule for Common Cold
  *Folium Isatidis* (isatis leaf　大青叶　*daqingye*)
  *Radix Isatidis* (isatis rot　板蓝根　*banlangen*)
  *Fructus Forsythiae* (forsythia fruit　连翘　*lianqiao*)
  *Rhizoma Bistortae* (bistort rhizome　拳参　*quanshen*)
  Mixed in proportion 2:2:1:1, and made into granule preparation, 18-36g, 3 times a day
  Actions: Remove fever and toxic elements.
  Indications: Upper respiratory infection, acute tonsillitis and pharyngitis.

Gexia Zhuyu Tang (　膈下逐瘀汤　) Decoction for Dissipating Blood Stasis Under the
Diaphragm
  *Radix Angelicae Sinensis* (Chinese angelica root　当归　*danggui*) 9g
  *Rhizoma Ligustici Chuanxiong* (chuanxiong rhizome　川芎　*chuanxiong*) 6g
  *Semen Persicae* (peach kernel　桃仁　*taoren*) 9g
  *Feces Trogopterorum* (trogopterus dung　五灵脂　*wulingzhi*) 6g
  *Cortex Moutan Radicis* (moutan bark　牡丹皮　*mudanpi*) 6g
  *Radix Paeoniae Rubra* (red peony root　赤芍　*chishao*) 6g
  *Radix Linderae* (lindera root　乌药　*wuyao*) 6g
  *Rhizoma Corydalis* (corydalis tuber　延胡索　*yanhusuo*) 3g
  *Radix Glycyrrhizae* (liquorice　甘草　*gancao*) 9g
  *Rhizoma Cyperi* (cyperus tuber　香附　*xiangfu*) 4.5g
  *Flos Carthami* (safflower　红花　*honghua*) 9g
  *Fructus Aurantii* (bitter orange　枳壳　*zhiqiao*) 4.5g
  Actions: Remove blood stasis, promote the flow of *qi* and relieve pain.
  Indications: Mass formation under the diaphragm with pain.

Gualou Xiebai Baijiu Tang (　瓜蒌薤白白酒汤　) Decoction of Trichosathes and Allium
with Wine
  *Fructus Trichosanthis* (trichosanthes fruit　瓜蒌　*gualou*) 15g
  *Bulbus Allii Macrostemi* (macrostem onion　薤白　*xiebai*) 9g
  *Vinum* (white wine) 30g
  Actions: Remove phlegm and promote the flow of *yang-qi*.
  Indications: Angina pectoris.

Guipi Tang (　归脾汤　) Decoction for Invigorating the Spleen and Nourishing the Heart
  *Radix Astragali* (astragalus root　黄芪　*huangqi*) 9g

*Rhizoma Atractylodis Macrocephalae* (white atractylodes rhizome  白术 *baizhu*) 9g

Poria (poria  茯苓 *fuling*) 9g

*Arillus Longan* (longan aril  龙眼肉 *longyanrou*) 9g

*Semen Ziziphi Spinosae* (wild jujuba seed  酸枣仁 *suanzaoren*) 9g

*Radix Codonopsis Pilosulae* (pilose asiabell root  党参 *dangshen*) 9g

*Radix Aucklandiae* (aucklandia root  木香 *muxiang*) 3g

*Radix Glycyrrhizae Praeparata* (prepared liquorice  炙甘草 *zhigancao*) 3g

*Radix Angelicae Sinensis* (Chinese angelica root  当归 *danggui*) 9g

*Radix Polygalae* (polygala root  远志 *yuanzhi*) 9g

Actions: Replenish *qi* and blood, invigorate the spleen and nourish the heart.

Indications: Weakness of both the spleen and heart, deficiency of *qi* and blood and bleeding due to failure of the spleen in keeping the blood circulating within the vessels.

Guizhi Fuzi Tang (  桂枝附子汤  ) Decoction of Cinnamon Twig and Aconite

*Ramulus Cinnamomi* (cinnamon twig  桂枝 *guizhi*) 12g

*Radix Aconiti Lateralis Praeparata* (prepared aconite root  附子 *fuzi*) 9g

*Rhizoma Zingiberis Recens* (fresh ginger  生姜 *shengjiang*) 9g

*Radix Glycyrrhizae Praeparata* (prepared liquorice  炙甘草 *zhigancao*) 6g

*Fructus Ziziphi Jujubae* (Chinese date  大枣 *dazao*) 6pcs

Actions: Remove cold, wind and damp to relieve rheumatic conditions.

Indications: Arthralgia with cold syndrome.

Haoqin Qingdan Tang (  蒿芩清胆汤  ) Sweet Wormwood and Scutellaria Decoction for Clearing Damp-heat from the Gallbladder

*Herba Artemisiae Annuae* (sweet wormwood  青蒿 *qinghao*) 6g

*Caulis Bambusae in Taeniam* (bamboo shavings  竹茹 *zhuru*) 9g

*Rhizoma Pinelliae* (prepared pinellia tuber  制半夏 *zhibanxia*) 4.5g

Poria (poria  茯苓 *fuling*) 9g

*Radix Scutellariae* (scutellaria root  黄芩 *huangqin*) 9g

*Fructus Aurantii* (bitter orange  枳壳 *zhiqiao*) 4.5g

*Pericarpium Citri Reticulatae* (tangerine peel  陈皮 *chenpi*) 4.5g

Green jade powder (containing talc powder, liquorice and natural indigo 碧玉散 *biyu san*) 9g

Actions: Remove heat and damp from the gallbladder, regulate the stomach and resolve phlegm.

Indications: Damp-heat and turbid phlegm in the gallbladder marked by chills and fever, bitterness in the mouth and distress in the hypochondriac region.

Huanglian Jiedu Tang (  黄连解毒汤  ) Antidotal Decoction of Coptis

*Rhizoma Coptidis* (coptis root  黄连 *huanglian*) 9g

*Radix Scutellariae* (scutellaria root  黄芩 *huangqin*) 6g

*Cortex Phellodendri* (phellodendron bark  黄柏 *huangbai*) 6g

*Fructus Gardeniae* (capejasmine fruit  栀子 *zhizi*) 9g

Actions: Remove intense heat and toxic elements.

Indications: High fever due to intense heat.

**Huangqi Jianzhong Tang** ( 黄芪建中汤 ) Decoction of Astragalus for Tonifying Middle-*jiao*

*Xiao Jianzhong Tang* (Minor Decoction for Strengthening Middle-*jiao*) plus *Radix Astragali* (astragalus root 黄芪 *huangqi*)

Actions: Warm and tonify the spleen and stomach.

Indications: Gastralgia and abdominal pain of deficiency-cold type as occurring in petic ulcer and chronic gastritis.

**Huangtu Tang** ( 黄土汤 ) Decoction of Baked Yellow Earth

Baked yellow earth ( 灶心土 *zaoxintu*) 30g

*Radix Rehmanniae* (dried rehmannia root 生地黄 *shengdihuang*) 9g

*Rhizoma Atractylodis Macrocephalae* (white atractylodes rhizome 白术 *baizhu*) 9g

*Radix Aconiti Lateralis Praeparata* (prepared aconite root 附子 *fuzi*) 9g

*Colla Corii Asini* (ass-hide glue 阿胶 *ejiao*) 9g

*Radix Scutellariae* (scutellaria root 黄芩 *huangqin*) 9g

*Radix Glycyrrhizae* (liquorice 甘草 *gancao*) 9g

Actions: Arrest bleeding by invigorating the spleen.

Indications: Bleeding due to failure of the spleen in keeping the blood circulating within the vessels.

**Huoxiang Zhengqi San** ( 藿香正气散 ) Powder of Asgastachis for Restoring Health

*Herba Agastachis* (agastache 藿香 *huoxiang*) 90g

*Folium Perillae* (perilla leaf 紫苏叶 *zisuye*) 30g

*Radix Angelicae Dahuricae* (dahurian angelica root 白芷 *baizhi*) 30g

*Pericarpium Arecae* (areca peel 大腹皮 *dafupi*) 30g

*Poria* (poria 茯苓 *fuling*) 30g

*Rhizoma Atractylodis Macrocephalae* (white atractylodes rhizome 白术 *baizhu*) 60g

*Rhizoma Pinelliae* (prepared pinellia tuber 制半夏 *zhibanxia*) 60g

*Pericarpium Citri Reticulatae* (tangerine peel 陈皮 *chenpi*) 60g

*Cortex Magnoliae Officinalis* (magnolia bark 厚朴 *houpo*) 60g

*Radix Platycodi* (platycodon root 桔梗 *jiegeng*) 60g

*Radix Glycyrrhizae* (liquorice 甘草 *gancao*) 75g

Mixed and made into powder, 6-9g for each dose to be taken with fresh ginger and Chinese date decoction.

Actions: Resolve damp and dispel pathogenic factors from the exterior of the body.

Indications: Affection by wind and cold with accumulation of dampness in the interior.

**Jiaotai Wan** ( 交泰丸 ) Coordinating Pill

*Rhizoma Coptidis* (coptis root 黄连 *huanglian*)

*Cortex Cinnamomi* (cinnamom bark 肉桂 *rougui*)

Actions: Coordinate the heart and kidneys.

Mixed in the proportion of 2:1 or 3:1, and made into powder, 3g for each dose.

Indications: Insomnia and palpitations due to incoordination between the heart and the kidneys.

**Jing Fang Baidu San** ( 荆防败毒散 ) Antiphlogistic Powder of Schizonepeta and Ledebouriella

*Herba Schizonepetae* (schizonepeta 荆芥 *jingjie*) 9g
*Radix Ledebouriellae* (ledebouriella root 防风 *fangfeng*) 9g
*Radix Bupleuri* (bupleurum root 柴胡 *chaihu*) 9g
*Radix Peucedani* (hogfennel root 前胡 *qianhu*) 9g
*Rhizoma Ligustici Chuanxiong* (chuanxiong rhizome 川芎 *chuanxiong*) 9g
*Fructus Aurantii* (bitter orange 枳壳 *zhiqiao*) 9g
*Rhizoma seu Radix Notopterygii* (notopterygium root 羌活 *qianghuo*) 9g
*Radix Angelicae Pubescentis* (pubescent angelica root 独活 *duhuo*) 9g
Poria (poria 茯苓 *fuling*) 9g
*Radix Platycodi* (platycodon root 桔梗 *jiegeng*) 9g
*Radix Glycyrrhizae* (liquorice 甘草 *gancao*) 4.5g
Actions: Cause diaphoresis and dispel wind and dampness.
Indications: Common cold affected by wind, cold and damp.

**Jinlingzi San** ( 金铃子散 ) Sichuan Chinaberry Powder

*Fructus Meliae Toosendan* (Sichuan chinaberry 金铃子 *jinlingzi*, also called 川楝子 *chuanlianzi*)
*Rhizoma Corydalis* (corydalis tuber 延胡索 *yanhusuo*)
Equal quantities, mixed and pulverized, 6-9g for each dose.
Actions: Promote the flow of *qi* in the liver and relieve pain.
Indications: hypochondriac pain caused by depression of the liver *qi*.

**Jinsuo Gujing Wan** ( 金锁固精丸 ) Golden Lock Pill for Maintaining the Kidney Essence

*Semen Astragali Complanati* (flattened milkvetch seed 沙苑蒺藜 *shayuanjili*) 60g
*Semen Euryales* (euryale seed 芡实 *qianshi*) 60g
*Stamen Nelumbinis* (lotus stamen 莲须 *lianxu*) 60g
*Os Draconis* (dragons's bone 龙骨 *longgu*) 30g
*Concha Ostreae* (oyster shell 牡蛎 *muli*) 30g
Pulverized, mixed and made into boluses, 1 bolus (9g) two or three times daily.
Actions: Consolidate the kidneys, arrest seminal emissions.
Indications: Seminal emissions, spermatorrhea.

**Jisheng Shenqi Wan** ( 济生肾气丸 ) Life-preserving Pill for Invigorating the Kidneys

*Radix Rehmanniae Praeparata* (prepared rehmannia root 熟地黄 *shudihuang*) 160g
*Fructus Corni* (dogwood fruit 山茱萸 *shanzhuyu*) 80g
*Rhizoma Discoreae* (Chinese yam 山药 *shanyao*) 80g
*Rhizoma Alismatis* (alismatis rhizome 泽泻 *zexie*) 60g
Poria (poria 茯苓 *fuling*) 120g
*Cortex Moutan Radicis* (moutan bark 牡丹皮 *mudanpi*) 60g
*Cortex Cinnamomi* (cinnamom bark 肉桂 *rougui*) 20g
*Radix Aconiti Lateralis Praeparata* (prepared aconite root 附子 *fuzi*) 20g
*Radix Achyranthis Bidentatae* (achyranthes root 牛膝 *niuxi*) 40g
*Semen Plantaginis* (plantain seed 车前子 *cheqianzi*) 40g
Mixed, pulverized, and made into pills, 6-9g 2-3 times daily.

Actions: Warm the kidneys and induce diuresis.
Indications: Edema or retained fluid due to deficiency kidney *yang*.

Liangfu Wan ( 良附丸 ) Galangal and Cyperus Pill
*Rhizoma Alpiniae Officinarum* (galangal rhizome 高良姜 *gaoliangjiang*)
*Rhizoma Cyperi* (cyperus tuber 香附 *xiangfu*)
Equal quantities, made into pills, 6g each dose.
Actions: Warm the stomach and regulate its *qi*.
Indications: Epigastric pain with distension and acid regurgitation.

Liu Junzi Tang [Wan] ( 六君子汤〔丸〕 ) Decoction [Pill] of Six Noble Ingredients
Si Junzi Tang (Decoction of Four Noble Drugs) plus *Rhizoma Pinelliae* (pinellia tuber 半夏 *banxia*) and *Pericarpium Citri Reticulatae* (tangerine peel 陈皮 *chenpi*)
Actions: Invigorate the spleen and stomach and remove damp-phlegm.
Indications: Weakness of the spleen and stomach complicated with damp-phlegm manifested as anorexia, loose bowels, cough with profuse thin expectoration, vomiting and acid regurgitation.

Liuwei Dihuang Wan ( 六味地黄丸 ) Bolus of Six Ingredients Including Rehmannia
*Radix Rehmanniae Praeparata* (prepared rehmannia root 熟地黄 *shudihuang*) 160g
*Fructus Corni* (dogwood fruit 山茱萸 *shanzhuyu*) 80g
*Rhizoma Dioscoreae* (Chinese yam 山药 *shanyao*) 80g
*Rhizoma Alismatis* (alismatis rhizome 泽泻 *zexie*) 60g
*Cortex Moutan Radicis* (moutan bark 牡丹皮 *mudanpi*) 60g
Poria (poria 茯苓 *fuling*) 60g
Mixed, pulverized and made into pills, 6-9g 2-3 times daily.
Actions: Replenish kidney *yin*.
Indications: Deficiency of kidney *yin* marked by dizziness, tinnitus, weakness of the loins and knees, seminal emissions, diabetes mellitus or consumptive fever.

Lizhong Tang ( 理中汤 ) Decoction for Regulating Middle-*jiao*
*Radix Codonopsis Pilosulae* (pilose asiabell root 党参 *dangshen*) 9g
*Rhizoma Zingiberis* (dried ginger 干姜 *ganjiang*) 6g
*Rhizoma Atractylodis Macrocephalae* (white atractylodes rhizome 白术 *baizhu*) 9g
*Radix Glycyrrhizae Praeparata* (prepared liquorice 炙甘草 *zhigancao*) 6g
Actions: Expel cold from the middle-*jiao* and invigorate the spleen.
Indications: Deficiency-cold of the spleen and stomach with anorexia, vomiting, diarrhea and abdominal pain.

Longdan Xiegan Tang ( 龙胆泻肝汤 ) Decoction of Gentian for Purging Liver Fire
*Radix Gentianae* (gentian root 龙胆草 *longdancao*) 12g
*Radix Bupleuri* (bupleurum root 柴胡 *chaihu*) 6g
*Rhizmoa Alismatis* (alismatis rhizome 泽泻 *zexie*) 9g
*Semen Plantaginis* (plantain seed 车前子 *cheqianzi*) 6g
*Caulis Clematidis Armandii* (Sichuan clematis stem 木通 *mutong*) 6g
*Radix Rehmanniae* (dried rehmannia root 生地黄 *shengdihuang*) 18g
*Radix Angelicae Sinensis* (Chinese angelica root 当归 *danggui*) 6g
*Fructus Gardeniae* (capejasmine fruit 栀子 *zhizi*) 9g

*Radix Scutellariae* (scutellaria root  黄芩  *huangqin*) 6g
*Radix Glycyrrhizae* (liquorice  甘草  *gancao*) 3g
Actions: Purge away fire and damp-heat from the liver and gallbladder meridians.
Indications: Fire or damp-heat in the liver and gallbladder meridians manifested as headache, hypochondriac pain and bitterness in the mouth or turbid urination and leukorrhagia, as occurring in hepatitis, cholecystitis, acute urinary infection, and acute pelvic inflammation.

Ma Xing Shi Gan Tang (  麻杏石甘汤  ) Decoction of Ephedra, Apricot Kernel, Gypsum and Liquorice
*Herba Ephedrae* (ephedra  麻黄  *mahuang*) 6g
*Semen Armenoiacae Amarum* (bitter apricot kernel  苦杏仁  *kuxingren*) 9g
*Gypsum Fibrosum* (gypsum  石膏  *shigao*) 24g
*Radix Glycyrrhizae* (liquorice  甘草  *gancao*) 6g
Actions: Clear the lungs of heat and relieve asthma.
Indications: Invasion of the lungs by heat.

Maiwei Dihuang Wan (  麦味地黄丸  ) Bolus of Rehmannia plus Ophiopogon and Schisandra
Liuwei Dihuang Wan (  六味地黄丸   Bolus of Six Ingredients Including *Rehmannia*) plus *Radix Ophiopogonis* (ophiopogon  麦冬  *maidong*) and *Fructus Schisandrae* (schisandra fruit  五味子  *wuweizi*)
Actions: Replenish *yin* of the lungs and kidneys.
Indications: Deficiency of *yin* of the lungs and kidneys.

Niuhuang Qingxin Wan (  牛黄清心丸  ) Bezoar Sedative Bolus
*Calculus Bovis* (cow-bezoar  牛黄  *niuhuang*)
*Cinnabaris* (cinnabar  朱砂  *zhusha*)
*Rhizoma Coptidis* (coptis root  黄连  *huanglian*)
*Radix Scutellariae* (scutellaria root  黄芩  *huangqin*)
*Fructus Gardeniae* (capejasmine fruit  栀子  *zhizi*)
*Radix Curcumae* (curcuma root  郁金  *yujin*)
Made into boluses, 3-6g twice a day
Actions: Remvoe toxic heat and induce sedation.
Indications: High fever with delirium and restlessness.

Pingwei San (  平胃散  ) Peptic Powder
*Rhizoma Atractylodis* (atractylodes rhizome  苍术  *cangzhu*) 9g
*Pericarpium Citri Reticulatae* (tangerine peel  陈皮  *chenpi*) 6g
*Cortex Magnoliae Officinalis* (magnolia bark  厚朴  *houpo*) 9g
*Radix Glycyrrhizae* (liquorice  甘草  *gancao*) 9g
Actions: Remove damp and invigorate the spleen and stomach.
Indications: Indigestion due to retention of damp in the spleen and stomach.

Qi Fu Tang (  芪附汤  ) Astragalus and Aconite Decoction
*Radix Astragali* (astragalus root  黄芪  *huangqi*) 6g
*Radix Aconiti Lateralis Praeparata* (prepared aconite root  附子  *fuzi*) 6g
*Rhizoma Zingiberis Recens* (fresh ginger  生姜  *shengjiang*) 10 slices

Actions: Replenish *yang-qi*.

Indications: Exhaustion of *yang-qi* with incessant sweating.

**Qiju Dihuang Wan** ( 杞菊地黄丸 ) Bolus of Rehmannia with Wolfberry and Chrysanthemum

Liuwei Dihuang Wan ( 六味地黄丸 Bolus of Six Ingredients Including *Rehmannia*) plus *Fructus Lycii* (wolfberry fruit 枸杞子 *gouqizi*) and *Flos Chrysanthemi* (chrysanthemum flower 菊花 *juhua*)

Actions: Replenish the kidneys and liver *yin*.

Indications: Deficiency of *yin* of the kidneys and liver manifested as dizziness, tinnitus, photophobia, lacrimination and blurred vision.

**Qingjin Huatan Tang** ( 清金化痰汤 ) Decoction for Clearing the Lungs and Resolving Phlegm

*Radix Scutellariae* (scutellaria root 黄芩 *huangqin*) 9g

*Fructus Gardeniae* (capejasmine fruit 栀子 *zhizi*) 9g

*Radix Ophiopogonis* (ophiopogon root 麦冬 *maidong*) 9g

*Rhizoma Anemarrhenae* (anemarrhena rhizome 知母 *zhimu*) 9g

*Radix Platycodi* (platycodon root 桔梗 *jiegeng*) 9g

*Cortex Mori Radicis* (mulberry bark 桑白皮 *sangbaipi*) 9g

*Bulbus Fritillariae Thunbergii* (thunberg fritillary bulb 浙贝母 *zhebeimu*) 9g

*Semen Trichosanthis* (trichosanthes seed 瓜蒌子 *gualouzi*) 9g

*Exocarpium* Citri Granis (pummelo peel 橘红 *juhong*) 9g

Poria (poria 茯苓 *fuling*) 9g

*Radix Glycyrrhiae* (liquorice 甘草 *gancao*) 3g

Actions: Clear the lungs of pathogenic heat, eliminate phlegm and relieve cough.

Indications: Bronchitis with cough due to phlegm-heat.

**Qingwei San** ( 清胃散 ) Powder for Clearing Stomach Fire

*Radix Angelicae Sinensis* (Chinese angelica root 当归 *danggui*) 6g

*Rhizoma Coptidis* (coptis root 黄连 *huanglian*) 5g

*Radix Rehmanniae* (dried rehmannia root 生地黄 *shengdihuang*) 12g

*Cortex Moutan Radicis* (moutan bark 牡丹皮 *mudanpi*) 6g

*Rhizoma Cimicifugae* (cimicifuga rhizome 升麻 *shengma*) 6g

Actions: Clear the stomach of pathogenic fire.

Indications: Excessive fire in the stomach.

**Qingwen Baidu Yin** ( 清瘟败毒饮 ) Antipyretic and Antitoxic Decoction

*Gypsum Fibrosum* (gypsum 石膏 *shigao*) 30-60g

*Radix Rehmanniae* (dried rehmannia root 生地黄 *shengdihuang*) 15-30g

*Cornu Rhinocerotis* (rhinoceros horn 犀角 *xijiao*) to be separately pulverized and taken after infusion 1-3g

*Rhizoma Coptidis* (coptis root 黄连 *huanglian*) 3-9g

*Fructus Gardeniae* (capejasmine fruit 栀子 *zhizi*) 6-12g

*Radix Platycodi* (platycodon root 桔梗 *jiegeng*) 3-6g

*Radix Scutellariae* (scutellaria root 黄芩 *huangqin*) 6-12g

*Rhizoma Anemarrhenae* (anemarrhena rhizome 知母 *zhimu*) 3-6g

*Radix Paeoniae Rubra* (red peony root　赤芍　*chishao*) 6-12g
*Fructus Forsythiae* (forsythia fruit　连翘　*lianqiao*) 6-12g
*Radix Scrophulariae* (scrophularia root　玄参　*xuanshen*) 6-12g
*Radix Glycyrrhizae* (liquorice　甘草　*gancao*) 3g
*Herba Lophatheri* (lophatherum　竹叶　*zhuye*) 3-6g
Actions: Remove intense heat and toxic substances from the *qi* and blood systems.
Indications: High fever, restlessness and delirium caused by intense heat in both *qi* and blood systems.

Qingying Tang (　清营汤　) Decoction for Clearing Heat in the *Ying* System
*Cornu Rhinocerotis* (rhinoceros horn　犀角　*xijiao*) to be separately pulverized and taken after infusion 2g
*Radix Rehmanniae* (dried rehmannia root　生地黄　*shengdihuang*) 15g
*Radix Scrophulariae* (scrophularia root　玄参　*xuanshen*) 9g
*Radix Ophiopogonis* (ophiopogon root　麦冬　*maidong*) 9g
*Flos Lonicerae* (honeysuckle flower　金银花　*jinyinhua*) 9g
*Fructus Forsythiae* (forsythia fruit　连翘　*lianqiao*) 6g
*Radix Salviae Miltiorrhizae* (red sage root　丹参　*danshen*) 6g
*Herba Lophatheri* (lophatherum　竹叶　*zhuye*) 3g
*Rhizoma Coptidis* (coptis root　黄连　*huanglian*) 5g
Actions: Clear away heat and toxic substances from the *ying* system.
Indications: High fever with delirium and skin eruption due to heat in the *ying* system.

Sangju Yin (　桑菊饮　) Decoction of Mulberry Leaf and Chrysanthemum
*Semen Armeniacae Amarum* (bitter apricot kernel　苦杏仁　*kuxingren*) 6g
*Fructus Forsythiae* (forsythia fruit　连翘　*lianqiao*) 6g
*Herba Menthae* (peppermint　薄荷　*bohe*) 3g
*Folium Mori* (mulberry leaf　桑叶　*sangye*) 8g
*Flow Chrysanthemi* (chrysanthemum flower　菊花　*juhua*) 6g
*Radix Platycodi* (platycodon root　桔梗　*jiegeng*) 6g
*Radix Glycyrrhizae* (liquorice　甘草　*gancao*) 6g
*Rhizoma Phragmitis* (reed rhizome　芦根　*lugen*) 3g
Actions: Dispel wind-heat and relieve cough.
Indications: Upper respiratory infection with cough and mild fever.

Sang Xing Tang (　桑杏汤　) Decoction of Mulberry Leaf and Apricot Kernel
*Semen Armenoiacae Amarum* (bitter apricot kernel　苦杏仁　*kuxingren*) 6g
*Folium Mori* (mulberry leaf　桑叶　*sangye*) 9g
*Radix Glehniae* (glehnia root　沙参　*shashen*) 12g
*Bulbus Fritillariae Thunbergii* (thunberg fritillary bulb　浙贝母　*zhebeimu*) 6g
*Semen Sojae Praeparata* (prepared soybean　淡豆豉　*dandouchi*) 6g
*Fructus Gardeniae* (capejasmine fruit　栀子　*zhizi*) 6g
*Pericarpium Piri* (pear peel　梨皮　*lipi*) 6g
Actions: Relieve dryness of the lungs.
Indications: Invasion of the lungs by dryness.

**Sanzi Tang** ( 三子汤 ) Decoction of Three Kinds of Seeds
   *Semen Sinapis Albae* (white mustard seed 白芥子 *baijiezi*) 6g
   *Fructus Perillae* (perilla seed 紫苏子 *zisuzi*) 9g
   *Semen Raphani* (radish seed 莱菔子 *laifuzi*) 9g
   Actions: Resolve phlegm and promote digestion.
   Indications: Cough and dyspnea with profuse expectoration, stuffiness in the chest and
   anorexia.

**Shaofu Zhuyu Tang** ( 少府逐瘀汤 ) Decoction for Removing Blood Stagnation in the
Lower Abdomen
   *Fructus Foeniculi* (common fennel fruit 小茴香 *xiaohuixiang*) 3g
   *Rhizoma Zingiberis* (dried ginger 干姜 *ganjiang*) 6g
   *Rhizoma Corydalis* (corydalis tuber 延胡索 *yanhusuo*) 9g
   *Myrrha* (myrrh 没药 *moyao*) 6g
   *Radix Angelicae Sinensis* (Chinese angelica root 当归 *danggui*) 6g
   *Rhizoma Ligustici Chuanxiong* (chuanxiong rhizome 川芎 *chuanxiong*) 6g
   *Cortex Cinnamomi* (cinnamon bark 肉桂 *rougui*) 3g
   *Radix Paeoniae Rubra* (red peony root 赤芍 *chishao*) 9g
   *Pollen Typhae* (cattail pollen 蒲黄 *puhuang*) 9g
   *Faeces Trogopterori* (trogopterus dung 五灵脂 *wulingzhi*) 9g
   Actions: Remove blood stasis, regulate menstruation and relieve pain.
   Indications: Mass in the lower abdomen, dysmenorrhea and menstrual disorders
   marked by discharge of dark coloured blood with clots.

**Shen Fu Tang** ( 参附汤 ) Decoction of Ginseng and Aconite
   *Radix Ginseng* (ginseng 人参 *renshen*) 12g
   *Radix Aconiti Lateralis Praeparata* (prepared aconite root 附子 *fuzi*) 9g
   Actions: Counteract shock.
   Indications: Shock.

**Shengmai San** ( 生脉散 ) Pulse-activating Powder
   *Radix Ginseng* (ginseng 人参 *renshen*) 10g
   *Radix Ophiopogonis* (ophiopogon root 麦冬 *maidong*) 15g
   *Fructus Schisandrae* (schisandra fruit 五味子 *wuweizi*) 6g
   Actions: Replenish *qi* and *yin*, and promote the production of body fluids.
   Indications: Impairment of *qi* and *yin* in febrile diseases, manifested by lassitude,
   excessive sweating, thirst, chronic cough with scanty expectoration, shortness of breath
   and palpitations, collapse and cardiogenic shock.

**Shen Ling Baizhu San** ( 参苓白术散 ) Powder of Ginseng, Poria and White Atracty-
lodes
   *Radix Ginseng* (ginseng 人参 *renshen*) 100g
   *Rhizoma Atractylodis Macrocephalae* (white atractylodes rhizome 白术 *baizhu*)
   100g
   *Poria* (poria 茯苓 *fuling*) 100g
   *Radix Glycyrrhizae* (liquorice 甘草 *gancao*) 100g
   *Rhizoma Dioscoreae* (Chinese yam 山药 *shanyao*) 100g

*Semen Dolichoris Album* (white hyacinth bean  白扁豆  *baibiandou*) 75g
*Semen Nelumbinis* (lotus seed  莲子  *lianzi*) 50g
*Semen Coicis* (coix seed  薏苡仁  *yiyiren*) 50g
*Fructus Amomi* (amomum fruit  砂仁  *sharen*) 50g
*Radix Platycodi* (platycodon rot  桔梗  *jiegeng*) 50g
Mixed and pulverized into powder, 6g each dose.
Actions: Replenish spleen *qi*, regulate the stomach and remove damp.
Indications: Deficiency of *qi* of the spleen and stomach accompanied by damp,
manifested as loss of appetite, abdominal distension and lassitude.

Shenqi Wan (  肾气丸  ) Bolus for Tonifying Kidney *Qi*
*Radix Rehmanniae* (dried rehmannia root  地黄  *dihuang*) 24g
*Fructus Corni* (dogwood fruit  山茱萸  *shanzhuyu*) 12g
*Rhizoma Dioscoreae* (Chinese yam  山药  *shanyao*) 12g
*Rhizoma Alismatis* (alismatis rhizome  泽泻  *zexie*) 9g
Poria (poria  茯苓  *fuling*) 9g
*Cortex Moutan Radicis* (moutan bark  牡丹皮  *mudanpi*) 9g
*Ramulus Cinnamomi* (cinnamom twig  桂枝  *guizhi*) 3g
*Radix Aconiti Lateralis Praeparata* (prepared aconite root  附子  *fuzi*) 3g
Mixed, pulverized and made into pills, 6-9g twice daily.
Actions: Warm and tonify kidney *yang*.
Indications: deficiency of kidney *yang* marked by aching and weakness of the loins
and knees, cold limbs, oliguria with edema or polyuria, cough and dyspnea, as
occurring in chronic nephritis, diabetes mellitus, diabetes insipitus and pulmonary
emphysema.

Shen Su Yin (  参苏饮  ) Ginseng and Perilla Drink
*Radix Ginseng* (ginseng  人参  *renshen*) 24g
*Folium Perillae* (perilla leaf  紫苏叶  *zisuye*) 24g
*Radix Puerariae* (pueraria root  葛根  *gegen*) 24g
*Radix Peucedani* (hogfennel root  前胡  *qianhu*) 24g
*Rhizoma Pinelliae* (pinellia tuber  半夏  *banxia*) 24g
Poria (poria  茯苓  *fuling*) 24g
*Pericarpium Citri Reticulatae* (tangerine peel  陈皮  *chenpi*) 15g
*Radix Glycyrrhizae* (liquorice  甘草  *gancao*) 15g
*Radix Platycodi* (platycodon root  桔梗  *jiegeng*) 15g
*Fructus Aurantii* (bitter orange  枳壳  *zhiqiao*) 15g
*Radix Aucklandiae* (aucklandia root  木香  *muxiang*) 15g
Mixed and pulverized into powder, 12g each dose, to be decocted with fresh ginger
and Chinese date.
Actions: Induce diaphoresis and resolve phlegm.
Indications: Common cold in patients with weak constitutions and accumulation of
phlegm, manifested by fever and chilliness with no sweat, headache, cough with viscid
expectoration and weak pulse.

Shihui San (  十灰散  ) Powder of Ashes of Ten Drugs
*Herba seu Radix Cirsii Japonici* (Japanese thistle  大蓟  *daji*)

*Herba Cephalanoploris* (field thistle 小蓟 *xiaoji*)
*Cacumen Biotae* (biota tops 侧柏叶 *cebaiye*)
*Radix Rubiae* (rubia root 茜草 *qiancao*)
*Radix et Rhizoma Rhei* (rhubarb 大黄 *dahuang*)
*Fructus Gardeniae* (capejasmine fruit 栀子 *zhizi*)
*Cortex Trachycarpi* (palm bark 棕榈皮 *zonglupi*)
*Cortex Moutan Radicis* (moutan bark 牡丹皮 *mudanpi*)
*Folium Nelumbinis* (lotus leaf 荷叶 *heye*)
*Rhizoma Imperatae* (cogongrass rhizome 白茅根 *baimaogen*)
Exqual quantities, broiled to charring and pulverized, 9-15g each dose.
Actions: Arrest bleeding by cooling the blood.
Indications: Various bleeding (such as hematemesis, hemoptysis and epistaxis) due to heat in the blood.

Shixiao San ( 失笑散 ) Wonderful Powder for Relieving Blood Stagnation
*Pollen Typhae* (cattail pollen 蒲黄 *puhuang*)
*Faeces Trogopterori* (trogopterus dung 五灵脂 *wulingzhi*)
Equal quantities, mixed and made into fine powder, 6g each dose.
Actions: Remove blood stasis and relieve pain.
Indications: Abdominal pain due to blood stasis and dysmenorrhea.

Si Junzi Tang ( 四君子汤 ) Decoction of Four Noble Drugs
*Radix Ginseng* (ginseng 人参 *renshen*) 12g
*Rhizoma Atractylodis Macrocephalae* (white atractylodes rhizome 白术 *baizhu*) 9g
*Poria* (poria 茯苓 *fuling*) 9g
*Radix Glycyrrhizae* (liquorice 甘草 *gancao*) 5g
Actions: Replenish *qi* and invigorate the spleen.
Indications: Deficiency of *qi* of the spleen and stomach.

Sini San ( 四逆散 ) Powder for Treating Cold Limbs
*Radix Bupleuri* (bupleurum root 柴胡 *chaihu*)
*Radix Paeoniae Alba* (white peony root 白芍 *baishao*)
*Fructus Aurantii Immaturus* (immature bitter orange 枳实 *zhishi*)
*Radix Glycyrrhizae Praeparata* (prepared liquorice 炙甘草 *zhigancao*)
Equal quantities, mixed and made into powder, 9-12g each dose.
Actions: Relieve stagnated heat and regulate the liver and spleen.
Indications: Syncope due to stagnation of heat in the interior, epigastric pain or diarrhea with tenesmus when the pulse is taut.

Sini Tang ( 四逆汤 ) Decoction for Resuscitation
*Radix Glycyrrhizae Praeparata* (prepared liquorice 炙甘草 *zhigancao*) 12g
*Rhizoma Zingiberis* (dried ginger 干姜 *ganjiang*) 9g
*Radix Aconiti Lateralis Praeparata* (prepared aconite root 附子 *fuzi*) 9g
Actions: Counteract collapse or shock.
Indications: Collapse, shock

Sishen Wan ( 四神丸 ) Pill of Four Miraculous Drugs
*Semen Myristicae* (nutmeg 肉豆蔻 *roudoukou*) 200g

*Fructus Psoraleae* (psoralea fruit  补骨脂  *buguzhi*) 400g
*Fructus Schisandrae* (schisandra fruit  五味子  *wuweizi*) 200g
*Fructus Evodiae* (evodia fruit  吴茱萸  *wuzhuyu*) 100g
Mixed, pulverized and made into pill, together with Chinese dates (200g) and the juice of 200g of fresh ginger, 6-9g twice daily.
Actions: Relieve diarrhea by warming the kidneys and spleen.
Indications: Chronic diarrhea due to deficiency-cold of the kidneys and the spleen.

Siwu Tang (　四物汤　) Decoction of Four Ingredients
*Radix Rehmanniae Praeparata* (prepared rehmannia root  熟地黄  *shudihuang*) 12g
*Radix Angelicae Sinensis* (Chinese angelica root  当归  *danggui*) 9g
*Rhizoma Ligustici Chuanxiong* (chuanxiong rhizome  川芎  *chuanxiong*) 6g
*Radix Paeoniae* (peony root  芍药  *shaoyao*) 9g
Actions: Replenish blood and regulate menstruation.
Indications: Deficiency of blood and menstrual disorders.

Suoquan Wan (　缩泉丸　) Pill for Reducing Urination
*Radix Linderae* (lindera root  乌药  *wuyao*)
*Fructus Alpiniae Oxyphyllae* (bitter cardamon  益智仁  *yizhiren*)
Equal quantities, mixed, pulverized and made into pills, 6g each dose.
Actions: Strengthen the kidneys to control urination.
Indications: Enuresis or frequent urination due to hypofunction of the kidneys.

Tianma Gouteng Yin (　天麻钩藤饮　) Decoction of Gastrodia and Uncaria
*Rhizoma Gastrodiae* (gastrodia tuber  天麻  *tianma*) 9g
*Ramulus Uncariae cum Uncis* (uncaria stem with hooks  钩藤  *gouteng*) 9g
*Concha Haliotidis* (abalones shell  石决明  *shijueming*) 30g
*Fructus Gardeniae* (capejasmine fruit  栀子  *zhizi*) 9g
*Radix Scutellariae* (scutellaria root  黄芩  *huangqin*) 9g
*Radix Cyathulae* (cyathula root  川牛膝  *chuanniuxi*) 9g
*Cortex Eucommiae* (eucommia bark  杜仲  *duzhong*) 9g
Poria (poria  茯苓  *fuling*) 9g
*Herba Leonuri* (motherwort  益母草  *yimucao*) 9g
*Ramulus Loranthi* (loranthus mulberry mistletoe  桑寄生  *sangjisheng*) 9g
*Caulis Polygoni Multiflori* (fleece-flower stem  首乌藤  *shouwuteng*) 15g
Actions: Subdue liver *yang*, nourish *yin* and reduce fire.
Indications: Syndrome of liver fire and wind due to deficiency of *yin* with exuberance of *yang*, marked by headache, dizziness, tinnitus, bitterness in the mouth, palpitations and insomnia, as often occurring in hypertension.

Tianwang Buxin Dan (　天王补心丹　) Cardiotonic Pill
*Radix Salviae Miltiorrhizae* (red sage root  丹参  *danshen*) 25g
*Rhizoma Acori Graminei* (grass-leaved sweetflag rhizome  石菖蒲  *shichangpu*) 25g
*Radix Codonopsis Pilosulae* (pilose asiabell root  党参  *dangshen*) 25g
*Semen Biotae* (arborvitae seed  柏子仁  *baiziren*) 50g
*Radix Ophiopogonis* (ophiopogon root  麦冬  *maidong*) 50g
*Radix Asparagi* (asparagus root  天冬  *tiandong*) 50g

*Radix Scrophulariae* (scrophularia root 玄参 *xuanshen*) 25g
*Fructus Schisandrae* (schisandra fruit 五味子 *wuweizi*) 50g
*Radix Rehmanniae* (dried rehmannia root 生地黄 *shengdihuang*) 200g
*Radix Angelicae Sinensis* (Chinese angelica root 当归 *danggui*) 50g
Poria (poria 茯苓 *fuling*) 25g
*Radix Polygalae* (polygala root 远志 *yuanzhi*) 25g
*Radix Platycodi* (platycodon root 桔梗 *jiegeng*) 25g
*Semen Ziziphi Spinosae* (wild jujuba seed 酸枣仁 *suanzaoren*) 50g
*Radix Glycyrrhizae* (liquorice 甘草 *gancao*) 25g
*Cinnabaris* (cinnabar 朱砂 *zhusha*) 10g
Pulverized, mixed and made into pills, 6g twice daily.
Actions: Replenish *yin* and blood and induce tranquilization.
Indications: Deficiency of heart *yin*, marked by palpitations, forgetfulness, insomnia and constipation.

Tongxie Yaofang ( 痛泻要方 ) Prescription of Importance for Diarrhea with Pain
*Radix Ledebouriellae* (ledebouriella root 防风 *fangfeng*) 6g
*Radix Atractylodis Macrocephalae* (white atractylodes rhizome 白术 *baizhu*) 9g
*Radix Paeoniae Alba* (white peony root 白芍 *baishao*) 9g
*Pericarpium Citri Reticulatae* (tangerine peel 陈皮 *chenpi*) 6g
Actions: Regulate the liver and the spleen.
Indications: Disorders of the liver and the spleen, marked by borborygmi and diarrhea accompanied by abdominal pain which is alleviated after bowel movement, as occurring in chronic colitis and irritable colon.

Wuling San ( 五苓散 ) Five Drugs Powder
*Polyporus Umbellatus* (umbellate pore-fungus 猪苓 *zhuling*) 9g
*Rhizoma Alismatis* (alismatis rhizome 泽泻 *zexie*) 9g
*Rhizomae Atractylodis Macrocephalae* (white atractylodes rhizome 白术 *baizhu*) 9g
Poria (poria 茯苓 *fuling*) 9g
*Ramulus Cinnamomi* (cinnamon twig 桂枝 *guizhi*) 6g
Actions: Promote diuresis.
Indications: Oliguria and edema.

Wupi Yin ( 五皮饮 ) Decoction of Peel of Five Drugs
*Cortex Zingiberis* (ginger peel 生姜皮 *shengjiangpi*) 6g
*Cortex Mori Radicis* (mulberry bark 桑白皮 *sangbaipi*) 9g
*Pericarpium Citri Reticulatae* (tangerine peel 陈皮 *chenpi*) 9g
*Pericarpium Arecae* (shell of areca nut 大腹皮 *dafupi*) 9g
Poria peel ( 茯苓皮 *fulingpi*) 24g
Actions: Induce diuresis.
Indications: Edema.

Xiangsha Liujunzi Tang ( 香砂六君子汤 ) Decoction of Aucklandia and Amomum with Six Noble Ingredients
Liu Junzi Tang ( 六君子汤 Decoction of Six Noble Ingredients) plus *Radix Aucklandiae* (aucklandia root 木香 *muxiang*) and *Fructus Amomi* (amomum fruit 砂仁

*sharen*).
Actions: Invigorate the spleen and stomach, regulate the flow of *qi* and remove damp.
Indications: Weakness of the spleen and stomach with stagnation of *qi* and damp.

Xiao Chaihu Tang (　小柴胡汤　) Minor Decoction of Bupleurum
   *Radix Bupleuri* (bupleurum root　柴胡　*chaihu*) 12g
   *Radix Scutellariae* (scutellaria root　黄芩　*huangqin*) 9g
   *Rhizoma Pinelliae* (pinellia tuber　半夏　*banxia*) 9g
   *Radix Codonopsis Pilosulae* (pilose asiabell root　党参　*dangshen*) 9g
   *Radix Glycyrrhizae Praeparata* (prepared liquorice　炙甘草　*zhigancao*) 6g
   *Rhizoma Zingiberis Recens* (fresh ginger　生姜　*shengjiang*) 9g
   *Fructus Ziziphi Jujubae* (Chinese date　大枣　*dazao*) 4pcs
   Actions: Treat *shaoyang* disease.
   Indications: *Shaoyang* disease characterized by alternate spells of chill and fever, distress and stuffy feeling in the chest, nausea, bitterness in the mouth and taut pulse, as occurring in pleuritis, malaria, pyelonephritis, acute cholecystitis and acute pancreatitis.

Xiao Jianzhong Tang (　小建中汤　) Minor Decoction for Strengthening Middle-*jiao*
   *Ramulus Cinnamomi* (cinnamon twig　桂枝　*guizhi*) 6g
   *Radix Paeoniae Alba* (white peony root　白芍　*baishao*) 12g
   *Radix Glycyrrhizae Praeparata* (prepared liquorice　炙甘草　*zhigancao*) 3g
   *Rhizoma Zingiberis Recens* (fresh ginger　生姜　*shengjiang*) 9g
   *Fructus Ziziphi Jujubae* (Chinese date　大枣　*dazao*) 4pcs
   *Saccharum Granorum* (malt extract　饴糖　*yitang*) 18g
   Actions: Warm and tonify the spleen and stomach and relieve spasmodic pain.
   Indications: Epigastric pain due to deficiency-cold of the spleen and stomach, as occurring in peptic ulcer.

Xiao Qinglong Tang (　小青龙汤　) Minor Decoction of Green Dragon
   *Herba Ephedrae* (ephedra　麻黄　*mahuang*) 6g
   *Radix Paeoniae* (peony root　芍药　*shaoyao*) 9g
   *Herba Asari* (asarum herb　细辛　*xixin*) 3g
   *Rhizoma Zingiberis* (dried ginger　干姜　*ganjiang*) 3g
   *Radix Glycyrrhizae Praeparata* (prepared liquorice　炙甘草　*zhigancao*) 3g
   *Ramulus Cinnamomi* (cinnamon twig　桂枝　*guizhi*) 3g
   *Fructus Schisandrae* (schisandra fruit　五味子　*wuweizi*) 6g
   *Rhizoma Pinelliae* (pinellia tuber　半夏　*banxia*) 9g
   Actions: Dispel cold from the exterior of the body, warm the lungs and resólve retained fluid.
   Indications: Affection by cold and wind with fluid retained in the interior, manifested as chilliness and fever without sweating, stuffiness in the chest, cough and asthma.

Xiao Xianxiong Tang (　小陷胸汤　) Minor Decoction for Relieving Stuffiness in the Chest
   *Rhizoma Coptidis* (coptis root　黄连　*huanglian*) 6g
   *Rhizoma Pinelliae* (pinellia tuber　半夏　*banxia*) 9g

*Fructus Trichosanthis* (trichosanthes fruit 瓜蒌 *gualou*) 30g
Actions: Remove heat and phlegm and relieve stuffiness in the chest.
Indications: Accumulation of heat and phlegm in the chest.

Xiaoyao San ( 逍遥散 ) Ease Powder
*Radix Glycyrrhizae Praeparata* (prepared liquorice 炙甘草 *zhigancao*) 15g
*Radix Angelicae Sinensis* (Chinese angelica root 当归 *danggui*) 30g
Poria (poria 茯苓 *fuling*) 30g
*Radix Paeoniae Alba* (white peony root 白芍 *baishao*) 30g
*Radix Atractylodis Macrocephalae* (white atractylodes rhizome 白术 *baizhu*) 30g
*Radix Bupleuri* (buplerum root 柴胡 *chaihu*) 30g
Mixed and made into powder, 6-9g each dose, to be taken with appropriate amount of
ginger and peppermint decoction.
Actions: Soothe the liver and strengthen the spleen.
Indications: Depression of liver *qi* with involvement of the spleen.

Xiexin Tang ( 泻心汤 ) Decoctions for Removing Heart-fire
*Radix et Rhizoma Rhei* (rhubarb 大黄 *dahuang*) 9g
*Rhizoma Coptidis* (coptis root 黄连 *huanglian*) 6g
*Radix Scutellariae* (scutellaria root 黄芩 *huangqin*) 9g
Actions: Purge away fire, remove toxic heat and damp.
Indications: Fire syndromes of excess type.

Xijiao Dihuang Tang ( 犀角地黄汤 ) Decoction of Rhinoceros Horn and Rehmannia
*Cornu Rhinocerotis* (rhinoceros horn 犀角 *xijiao*) to be separately pulverized and
taken after infusion 1.5-3g
*Radix Rehmanniae* (dried rehmannia root 生地黄 *shengdihuang*) 30g
*Radix Paeoniae Rubra* (red peony root 赤芍 *chishao*) 12g
*Cortex Moutan Radicis* (moutan bark 牡丹皮 *mudanpi*) 9g
Actions: Remove toxic heat from the blood and eliminate blood stasis.
Indications: Fever with delirium and eruption or hematemesis, epistaxis and hemato-
chezia due to heat in the blood.

Xing Su San ( 杏苏散 ) Apricot Kernel and Perilla Powder
*Folium Perillae* (perilla leaf 紫苏叶 *zisuye*) 6g
*Semen Armenoiacae Amarum* (bitter apricot kernel 苦杏仁 *kuxingren*) 9g
*Rhizoma Zingiberis Recens* (fresh ginger 生姜 *shengjiang*) 6g
*Radix Platycodi* (platycodon root 桔梗 *jiegeng*) 6g
Poria (poria 茯苓 *fuling*) 6g
*Rhizoma Pinelliae* (pinellia tuber 半夏 *banxia*) 3g
*Radix Glycyrrhizae* (liquorice 甘草 *gancao*) 3g
*Peucedanum* (hogfennel root 前胡 *qianhu*) 9g
*Pericarpium Citri Reticulatae* (tangerine peel 陈皮 *chenpi*) 6g
*Fructus Aurantii* (bitter orange 枳壳 *zhiqiao*) 6g
*Fructus Ziziphi Jujubae* (Chinese date 大枣 *dazao*) 2pcs
Actions: Dispel wind-cold and relieve cough.
Indications: Invasion of the lungs by wind-cold.

**Xuefu Zhuyu Tang** ( 血府逐瘀汤 ) Decotion for Removing Blood Stasis in the Chest
*Radix Angelicae Sinensis* (Chinese angelica root 当归 *danggui*) 9g
*Radix Rehmanniae* (dried rehmannia root 生地黄 *shengdihuang*) 9g
*Semen Persicae* (peach kernel 桃仁 *taoren*) 12g
*Flos Carthami* (safflower 红花 *honghua*) 9g
*Fructus Aurantii* (bitter orange 枳壳 *zhiqiao*) 6g
*Radix Paeoniae Rubra* (red peony root 赤芍 *chishao*) 6g
*Radix Bupleuri* (bupleurum root 柴胡 *chaihu*) 3g
*Radix Glycyrrhizae* (liquorice 甘草 *gancao*) 3g
*Rhizoma Ligustici Chuanxiong* (chuanxiong rhizome 川芎 *chuanxiong*) 5g
*Radix Platycodi* (platycodon root 桔梗 *jiegeng*) 5g
*Radix Achyranthis Bidentatae* (achyranthes root 牛膝 *niuxi*) 9g
Actions: Remove blood stasis, promote the flow of *qi* and relieve pain.
Indications: Blood stasis associated with stagnation of liver *qi*, manifested as persistent chest or hypochondriac pain, stubborn headache, palpitations, insomnia and irritability.

**Yangxin Tang** ( 养心汤 ) Decoction for Nourishing the Heart
*Radix Astragali* (astragalus root 黄芪 *huangqi*) 5g
*Poria cum Radice Pino* (sclerotium of poria with pine root 茯神 *fushen*) 5g
Poria (poria 茯苓 *fuling*) 5g
*Rhizoma Pinelliae Fermenatatae* (fermented pinellia tuber 半夏曲 *banxiaqu*) 5g
*Radix Angelicae Sinensis* (Chinese angelica root 当归 *danggui*) 5g
*Rhizome Ligustici Chuanxiong* (chuanxiong rhizome 川芎 *chuanxiong*) 5g
*Radix Polygalae* (polygala root 远志 *yuanzhi*) 3g
*Semen Ziziphae Spinosae* (wild jujuba seed 酸枣仁 *suanzaoren*) 3g
*Cortex Cinnamomi* (cinnamom bark 肉桂 *rougui*) 3g
*Semen Biotae* (arborvitae seed 柏子仁 *baiziren*) 3g
*Fructus Schisandrae* (schisandra fruit 五味子 *wuweizi*) 3g
*Radix Genseng* (ginseng 人参 *renshen*) 3g
*Radix Glycyrrhizae Praeparata* (prepared liquorice 炙甘草 *zhigancao*) 1.5g
Actions: Replenish *qi* and blood, nourish the heart and induce tranquilization.
Indications: Deficiency of *qi* and blood of the heart with insomnia and palpitations.

**Yiguan Jian** ( 一贯煎 ) Ever-effective Decoction for Nourishing the Liver and Kidneys
*Radix Glehniae* (glehnia root 北沙参 *beishashen*) 9g
*Radix Ophiopogonis* (ophiopogon root 麦冬 *maidong*) 9g
*Radix Angelicae Sinensis* (Chinese angelica root 当归 *danggui*) 18g
*Radix Rehmanniae* (dried rehmannia root 生地黄 *shengdihuang*) 9g
*Fructus Lycii* (wolfberry fruit 枸杞子 *gouqizi*) 9g
*Fructus Meliae Toosendan* (Sichuan chinaberry 川楝子 *chuanlianzi*) 9g
Actions: Replenish *yin* and regulate the liver.
Indications: Deficiency of *yin* of the liver and kidneys with stagnation of liver *qi*, marked by dizziness, aching of the loins, dryness of the throat, hypochondriac pain and distension and acid regurgitation, as occurring in chronic hepatitis and chronic gastritis.

**Yinchenhao Tang (** 茵陈蒿汤 **) Oriental Wormwood Decoction**
*Herba Artemisiae Scoporiae* (oriental wormwood  茵陈 *yinchen*) 30g
*Fructus Gardeniae* (capejasmine fruit  栀子 *zhizi*) 15g
*Radix et Rhizoma Rhei* (rhubarb  大黄 *dahuang*) 10g
Actions: Remove damp-heat.
Indications: Jaundice due to damp-heat, as occurring in acute icteric hepatitis.

**Yinchen Wuling San (** 茵陈五苓散 **) Powder of Oriental Wormwood and Five Drugs**
Wuling San (  五苓散  Five Drugs Powder) plus *Herba Artemisiae* (oriental worm-
wood 茵陈 *yinchen*)
Actions: Remove damp-heat.
Indications: Syndrome of damp-heat with more damp than heat.

**Yinchen Zhu Fu Tang (** 茵陈术附汤 **) Decoction of Oriental Wormwood, White Atrac-
tylodes and Aconite**
· *Herba Artemisiae Scoporiae* (oriental wormwood  茵陈 *yinchen*) 3g
*Rhizoma Atractylodis Macrocephalae* (white atractylodes rhizome 白术 *baizhu*)
6g
*Radix Aconiti Lateralis Praeparata* (prepared aconite root  附子 *fuzi*) 1.5g
*Riezoma Zingiberis* (dried ginger  干姜 *ganjiang*) 1.5g
*Radix Glycyrrhizae* (liquorice  甘草 *gancao*) 3g
*Cortex Cinnamomi* (cinnamom bark  肉桂 *rougui*) 1g
Actions: Warm the spleen, remove dampness and relieve jaundice.
Indications: *Yin*-jaundice caused by cold-dampness.

**Yinqiao Jiedu Wan [Pian] (** 银翘解毒丸[片] **) Antiphlogistic Bolus [Tablet] of Lonicera
and Forsythia**
Composition same as Yin Qiao San (  银翘散  Powder of Lonicera and Forsythia),
made into pills or tablets, 1 bolus (3g) or 4 tablets, 2-3 times a day.
Actions and indications: See Yin Qiao San.

**Yin Qiao San (** 银翘散 **) Powder of Lonicera and Forsythia**
*Fructus Forsythiae* (forsythia fruit  连翘 *lianqiao*) 30g
*Flos Lonicerae* (honeysuckle flower  金银花 *jinyinhua*) 30g
*Radix Platycodi* (platycodon root  桔梗 *jiegeng*) 18g
*Herba Menthae* (peppermint  薄荷 *bohe*) 18g
*Herba Lophatheri* (lophatherum  淡竹叶 *danzhuye*) 12g
*Radix Glycyrrhizae* (liquorice  甘草 *gancao*) 15g
*Herba Schizonepetae* (schizonepeta spike  荆芥穗 *jingjiesui*) 18g
*Semen Sojae Praeparatum* (prepared soybean  淡豆豉 *dandouchi*) 15g
*Fructus Arctii* (arctium fruit  牛蒡子 *niubangzi*) 18g
Mixed and pulverized into powder, each dose 20g of powder decocted with appropriate
quantity of *Rhizoma Phragmitis* (reed rhizome  芦根 *lugen*).
Actions: Dispel wind-heat and remove toxic elements.
Indications: Initial stage of epidemic febrile disease, manifested as fever with mild
chilliness, headache, thirst, cough, sore throat, reddened tongue tip, whitish or yellow-
ish tongue coating and floating and rapid pulse.

**Yiwei Tang** ( 益胃汤 ) Stomach-nourishing Decoction
*Radix Glehniae* (glehnia root  沙参  *shashen*) 9g
*Radix Ophiopogonis* (ophiopogon root  麦冬  *maidong*) 15g
Crystal Sugar ( 冰糖  *bingtang*) 3g
*Radix Rehmanniae* (dried rehmannia root  生地黄  *shengdihuang*) 15g
*Rhizoma Polygonati Odorati* (fragrant solomonseal rhizome 玉竹  *yuzhu*) 4.5g
Actions: Nourish the stomach and promote the production of body fluids.
Indications: Deficiency of stomach *yin*.

**Yougui Wan** ( 右归丸 ) Kidney-*yang* Reinforcing Bolus
*Radix Rehmanniae Praeparata* (prepared rehmannia root  熟地黄  *shudihuang*) 24g
*Fructus Corni* (dogwood fruit  山茱萸  *shanzhuyu*) 9g
*Rhizoma Discoreae* (Chinese yam  山药  *shanyao*) 12g
*Frutus Lycii* (wolfberry fruit  枸杞子  *gouqizi*) 12g
*Semen Cuscutae* (dodder seed  菟丝子  *tusizi*) 12g
*Colla Cornus Cervi* (antler glue  鹿角胶  *lujiaojiao*) 12g
*Cortex Eucommiae* (eucommia bark  杜仲  *duzhong*) 12g
*Radix Angelicae Sinensis* (Chinese angelica root  当归  *danggui*) 9g
*Cortex Cinnamomi* (cinnamom bark  肉桂  *rougui*) 6-12g
*Radix Aconiti Lateralis Praeparata* (prepared aconite root  附子  *fuzi*) 6-18g
Made into honeyed boluses, 9g twice daily.
Actions: Invigorate kindey *yang*.
Indications: Deficiency of kidney *yang*.

**Yougui Yin** ( 右归饮 ) Kidney-*yang* Reinforcing Decoction
*Radix Rehmanniae Praeparata* (prepared rehmannia root  熟地黄  *shudihuang*) 8-50g
 *Fructus Corni* (dogwood fruit  山茱萸  *shanzhuyu*) 3g
*Rhizoma Discoreae* (Chinese yam  山药  *shanyao*) 6g
*Fructus Lycii* (wolfberry fruit  枸杞子  *gouqizi*) 6g
*Radix Glycyrrhizae* (liquorice  甘草  *gancao*) 5g
*Cortex Eucommiae* (eucommia bark  杜仲  *duzhong*) 6g
*Cortex Cinnamomi* (cinnamom bark  肉桂  *rougui*) 4g
*Radix Aconiti Lateralis Praeparata* (prepared aconite root  附子  *fuzi*) 7g
Actions: Warm and reinforce the kidneys.
Indications: Deficiency of kidney *yang*.

**Yunü Jian** ( 玉女煎 ) Gypsum Decoction
*Gypsum Fibrosum* (gypsum  石膏  *shigao*) 15-30g
*Radix Rehmanniae Praeparata* (prepared rehmannia root  熟地黄  *shudihuang*) 15-30g
*Radix Ophiopogonis* (ophiopogon root  麦冬  *maidong*) 6g
*Rhizoma Anemarrhenae* (anemarrhena rhizome 知母*zhimu*) 4.5g
*Radix Achyranthis Bidentatae* (achyranthes root  牛膝  *niuxi*) 4.5g
Actions: Clear the stomach of fire and replenish *yin*.
Indications: Deficiency of stomach *yin* with excessive stoamch fire, marked by thirst, ulcers in the mouth, painful swollen gums and epistaxis, as occurring in diabetes mellitus.

**Yupingfeng San** ( 玉屏风散 ) Jade-screen Powder
*Radix Astragali* (astragalus root 黄芪 *huangqi*) 180g
*Rhizoma Atractylodis Macrocephalae* (white atractylodes rhizome 白术 *baizhu*) 60g
*Radix Ledebouriellae* (ledebouriella root 防风 *fangfeng*) 60g
Mixed and pulverized, 10g twice daily
*Actions*: Replenish *qi*, strengthen the superficial body resistance and arrest sweating.
Indications: Lowered body resistance with vulnerability to colds.

**Zengye Tang** ( 增液汤 ) Fluid-increasing Decoction
*Radix Scrophulariae* (scrophularia root 玄参 *xuanshen*) 30g
*Radix Ophiopogonis* (ophiopogon root 麦冬 *maidong*) 24g
*Radix Rehmanniae* (dried rehmannia root 生地黄 *shengdihuang*) 24g
Actions: Promote the production of body fluids.
Indications: Deficiency of body fluids in febrile diseases.

**Zhen'gan Xifeng Tang** ( 镇肝熄风汤 ) Decoction for Tranquilizing Liver-wind
*Radix Achyranthis Bidentatae* (achyranthes root 牛膝 *niuxi*) 30g
*Haematitum* (hematite 赭石 *zheshi*) 30g
*Os Draconis* (dragon's bone 龙骨 *longgu*) 15g
*Concha Ostreae* (oyster shell 牡蛎 *muli*) 15g
*Plastrum Testudinis* (tortoise plastron 龟板 *guiban*) 15g
*Radix Paeoniae Alba* (white peony root 白芍 *baishao*) 15g
*Radix Scrophulariae* (scrophularia root 玄参 *xuanshen*) 15g
*Radix Asparagi* (asparagus root 天冬 *tiandong*) 15g
*Fructus Meliae Toosendan* (Sichuan chinaberry 川楝子 *chuanlianzi*) 6g
*Fructus Hordei Germinatus* (germinated barley 麦芽 *maiya*) 6g
*Herba Artemisiae* (oriental wormwood 茵陈 *yinchen*) 6g
*Radix Glycyrrhizae* (liquorice 甘草 *gancao*) 4g
Actions: Subdue liver fire and calm the wind.
Indications: Exuberant liver fire with stirring-up of wind, manifested as vertigo and tinnitus, syncope or apoplexy.

**Zhenwu Tang** ( 真武汤 ) Decoction for Invigorating *Yang*
Poria (poria 茯苓 *fuling*) 9g
*Radix Paeoniae* (peony root 芍药 *shaoyao*) 9g
*Rhizoma Zingiberis Recens* (fresh ginger 生姜 *shengjiang*) 9g
*Rhizoma Atractylodis Macrocephalae* (white atractylodes rhizome 白术 *baizhu*) 6g
*Radix Aconiti Lateralis Praeparata* (prepared aconite root 附子 *fuzi*) 9g
Actions: Induce diuresis by warming the *yang* of the spleen and kidneys.
Indications: Edema due to deficiency of *yang* of the spleen and kidneys.

**Zuogui Wan** ( 左归丸 ) Kidney-*yin* Replenishing Bolus
*Radix Rehmanniae Praeparata* (prepared rehmannia root 熟地黄 *shudihuang*) 24g
*Fructus Corni* (dogwood fruit 山茱萸 *shanzhuyu*) 12g
*Rhizoma Dioscoreae* (Chinese yam 山药 *shanyao*) 12g
*Fructus Lycii* (wolfberry fruit 枸杞子 *gouqizi*) 12g
*Semen Cuscutae* (dodder seed 菟丝子 *tusizi*) 12g

*Radix Achyranthis Bidentatae* (achyranthes root  牛膝  *niuxi*) 9g
*Colla Cornus Cervi* (antler glue  鹿角胶  *lujiaojiao*) 12g
*Colla Plastri Testudinis* (tortoise-plastron glue  龟板胶  *guibanjiao*) 12g
Made into honeyed boluses, 9g twice daily.
Actions: Replenish kidney *yin*.
Indications: Deficiency of kidney *yin*.

**中医内科学**

谢竹藩、廖家桢　编著

\*

外文出版社出版

（中国北京百万庄路 24 号）

邮政编码 100037

北京外文印刷厂印刷

中国国际图书贸易总公司发行

（中国北京车公庄西路 35 号）

北京邮政信箱第 399 号　邮政编码 100044

1993 年（36 开）第一版

（英）

ISBN 7—119—01600—8 /R・96（外）

04070

14—E—2812S